How to Write Your Nursing Dissertation

T0201158

How to Write Your Nursing Dissertation

SECOND EDITION

Edited by

Alan Glasper
University of Southampton
Southampton, UK

Diane Carpenter
University of Plymouth
Truro, UK

WILEY Blackwell

This edition first published 2021
© 2021 John Wiley & Sons Ltd

Edition History
Wiley-Blackwell (1e, 2013)

Registered Offices
John Wiley & Sons, Inc., 111 River Street, Hoboken, NJ 07030, USA
John Wiley & Sons Ltd, The Atrium, Southern Gate, Chichester, West Sussex, PO19 8SQ, UK

Editorial Office
9600 Garsington Road, Oxford, OX4 2DQ, UK

For details of our global editorial offices, customer services, and more information about Wiley products visit us at www.wiley.com.

Wiley also publishes its books in a variety of electronic formats and by print-on-demand. Some content that appears in standard print versions of this book may not be available in other formats.

Library of Congress Cataloging-in-Publication Data
Names: Glasper, Edward Alan, editor. | Carpenter, Diane, editor.
Title: How to write your nursing dissertation / edited by Edward Alan
   Glasper, Diane Teresa Carpenter.
Description: Second edition. | Hoboken, NJ : Wiley-Blackwell, 2021. |
   Includes bibliographical references and index.
Identifiers: LCCN 2020030532 (print) | LCCN 2020030533 (ebook) | ISBN
   9781119757733 (paperback) | ISBN 9781119757740 (Adobe PDF) | ISBN
   9781119757757 (epub)
Subjects: MESH: Academic Dissertations as Topic | Evidence-Based Nursing |
   Writing | Nursing Research | United Kingdom
Classification: LCC R119 (print) | LCC R119 (ebook) | NLM WY 100.7 | DDC
   808.06/661–dc23
LC record available at https://lccn.loc.gov/2020030532
LC ebook record available at https://lccn.loc.gov/2020030533

Cover Design: Wiley
Cover Image: © TECHDESIGNWORK / iStockphoto

Set in 9.5/12pt Minion by SPi Global, Pondicherry, India
Printed and bound by CPI Group (UK) Ltd, Croydon, CR0 4YY

C9781119757733_240221

Contents

List of Contributors

Dr Justine Barksby
Senior Lecturer and Subject Lead for Learning Disabilities
Leicester School of Nursing and Midwifery
Faculty of Health and Life Sciences
De Montfort University
Leicester, UK

Megan Bonner-Janes
Lecturer in Child and Psychosocial Health
Faculty of Health Sciences
University of Southampton
Southampton, UK

Dr Diane Carpenter
Lecturer in Mental Health Nursing
School of Nursing and Midwifery (Faculty of Health)
University of Plymouth
Plymouth, UK

Dr Michelle Cowen
Director of Learning in Practice
Faculty of Health Sciences
University of Southampton
Southampton, UK

Dr Alan Glasper
Emeritus Professor of Nursing Studies
Faculty of Health Sciences
University of Southampton
Southampton, UK

Lisa Harding
University of Winchester
Winchester, UK

Dr Tracey Harding
Lecturer/Associate Head of School for Postgraduate Study
School of Nursing and Midwifery (Faculty of Health)
University of Plymouth
Plymouth, UK

Sarah Adrienne Hughes
University of Southampton
Southampton, UK

Dr Ellen Kitson-Reynolds
Principal Teaching Fellow
Midwifery Programmes Lead and Lead Midwife for Education
Faculty of Health Sciences
University of Southampton
Southampton, UK

Dr Andrée le May
Emeritus Professor, University of Southampton, Southampton;
Visiting Senior Fellow, Institute of Public Health, University of
Cambridge
Cambridge, UK

Dr Jane March-McDonald
Lecturer in Adult Nursing
School of Nursing and Midwifery (Faculty of Health)
University of Plymouth
Plymouth, UK

Mary O'Toole
Lecturer in Mental Health Nursing
School of Nursing and Midwifery (Faculty of Health)
University of Plymouth
Plymouth, UK

Foreword

Only 20 years ago, the idea that students should be taught about the evidence that underpins clinical practice was regarded as a dangerously radical one. This book shows how great the change over the intervening period has been. During that time small communities of researchers and methodologists have created alliances with practitioners and patients around specific clinical problems. They have subjected what is known about the clinical and cost-effectiveness of different treatments and modes of professional practice to rigorous tests, using primary studies, clinical trials, systematic reviews and meta-analyses. In almost every area of healthcare, the application of evidence has led to a revolution in the quality of care that patients receive.

This book is part of that revolution, and every chapter is written by practitioners with real-life experience of understanding and applying evidence. Each chapter is written in a way that emphasises its application to real-life problems. This is important because 'evidence' isn't an abstract problem. And it isn't just a problem for students either. Politicians, policy-makers and managers all struggle with evidence, and seek ways to make it meaningful to their own situations. Sometimes this means that evidence isn't always what it seems. My own research has shown how clinical trials of new health technologies are hard for their sponsors to fathom (May, 2006), and how policy-makers seek quite different kinds of evidence for their effectiveness that sometimes fit poorly with wider conceptions of robustness and rigour but very well with the interests and goals of organisations (May, 2007).

So, evidence is important because it offers a rational basis for the allocation of healthcare resources and the provision of patient care. But what is and isn't evidence isn't just a problem of method. Underpinning that problem is a deeper one, alluded to in almost every chapter in the book – but particularly in Diane Carpenter's chapter on historical methods and evidence – which is that what counts as evidence is sometimes contingent on time and place.

If evidence is important because it offers a rational basis for practice, it's worth remembering that much of what we see practiced every day in hospitals and clinics has no evidence base. The challenge for a new generation of students is to change that. This book will start to give you the tools to achieve that.

Carl May
Professor of Medical Sociology
London School of Hygiene and Tropical Medicine

May, C. (2006) Mobilizing modern facts: Health Technology Assessment and the politics of evidence. Sociology of Health and Illness, **28**, 513–532.
May, C. (2007) The clinical encounter and the problem of context. Sociology, **41**, 29–45.

Preface

This book provides the reader with a clear knowledge of the fundamental steps needed to write an evidence-based practice healthcare dissertation/ final project or evidence-informed decision-making assignment at foundation degree, degree or postgraduate level. It aims to bring together key ideas and concepts related to evidence-based practice and research use which is pertinent to the production of a dissertation/project or evidence-informed decision-making assignment. The book uses fabricated individual person scenarios that you, the reader, can identify with on your academic journey. It will demonstrate the way in which all the components of evidence-based healthcare, such as research use skills, standard setting, legal and ethical frameworks, audit and benchmarking, are drawn together for the purpose of writing a dissertation/project or evidence-informed decision-making assignment.

Primary target

The main audiences for this book are nursing and nursing associate students/ trainees and other healthcare students who are required to complete an evidence-based practice piece of work as part fulfilment of a foundation, honours or postgraduate master's degree.

Secondary target

This book will also be used by qualified healthcare personnel who require evidence-based care knowledge for their day-to-day clinical activities.

Style of the book

The book is written using a very clear and engaging scenario style. This has been used to provide a logical structure and progression to the ideas embodied within the text that readers will find relevant to their dissertation work.

We are confident that this book will provide you, the reader, with a clear knowledge of the fundamental aspects of evidence-based practice needed to write your healthcare dissertation/project or evidence-informed decision-making assignment and help provide you with the knowledge to deliver quality evidence-based care within current healthcare environments.

Alan Glasper and Diane Carpenter

About the companion website

This book is accompanied by a companion website:

www.wiley.com/go/glasper/nursingdissertation2e

The website includes:

- Five Bonus Chapters
- Frameworks and tools
- Dissertation
- Sample papers
- Writing for Publication

Scan this QR code to visit the companion website.

The Scenarios

Sue is a senior staff nurse who works in an elderly care unit of a large tertiary teaching hospital. She entered nursing late after having a family and completed her enhanced diploma in adult nursing four years earlier. Her ward manager has sponsored her to undertake a 'top-up degree' programme at her local university. The programme she has enrolled on is specially designed to allow enhanced/advanced diplomate holders to progress towards gaining an honours degree classification to bring their academic qualifications up to the standard of initial nurse training today. In essence, the course entails attending a number of taught study days, where she will learn about the nuts and bolts of understanding evidence-based practice. The assessment, if successfully completed, will confer upon her a degree classification that is based on the submission of a 10 000-word dissertation. Sue has not opened a textbook for nearly five years and although she tries to keep up to date by reading a nursing journal which her ward subscribes to, she is full of trepidation about the course she has enrolled on.

Her good friend and neighbour, Sam, aged 31, works in the local children's hospital as a ward manager. He is already a graduate, having completed a degree in children's nursing some 10 years ago. Sam, likewise, has been out of the studying habit for many years. He is now seeking to become a clinical nurse specialist and has been fortunate to receive funding from his hospital to undertake an MSc in Nursing at the same university as Sue. Sam has a 'learning difference' and is dyslexic. The dissertation element of the MSc programme is similar to the undergraduate dissertation; it is in the format of a critical review of the evidence base for practice but this time is 20 000 words in length. Sam is equally worried about completing the dissertation element of the course.

Alisha left school without taking A-levels; she sought employment as a healthcare assistant at her local NHS Trust. Her ward managers recognised that Alisha had potential and when the new Nursing Associate Foundation Degree by the local university was launched in 2018 they sponsored her to undertake this new course. Alisha is now in her second and final year and is looking forward to registering with the Nursing and Midwifery Council as a qualified Nursing Associate. She must successfully complete an evidence-based practice project of 4000 words before completing the course. She and her friend Charlotte, who is a third-year student nurse, often meet in the library.

Charlotte is a third-year undergraduate student nurse and has been recently assessed as having a learning difference. She has been having regular support meetings with the faculty learning support manager. She has to write a 7000-word evidence-based practice assignment based on a topic of interest arising from her clinical placement experience.

Scenario 1: Starting the dissertation journey

Sue and Sam are facing the next challenge in their academic journey – the writing and completion of a dissertation. There is something about the dissertation that unsettles the two friends, which might be related to the size of the assignment or the freedom in choosing a project title. In reality, the dissertation gives them great freedom to choose what excites them as professionals working in clinical domains, but there are some principles that each will have to follow in developing their ideas. Charlotte and Alisha have been advised to reflect on their clinical experience to date to help them identify either gaps in their knowledge or occasions when they have become aware of different approaches to care for patients with similar conditions. They are reminded that the purpose of evidence-based practice is to ensure that clinical decisions are based on the best, most reliable evidence.

Scenario 2: Sourcing and accessing evidence for your dissertation

Sue asks Sam for advice. She has some ideal 'evidence' for her dissertation but it is from a Sunday supplement magazine; does this count as evidence, she asks? Sam tells her about the work of Professor Andrée le May. Charlotte, despite having learned the principles of searching electronic databases in her first year, has not been very adventurous with this since and has tended to rely on one database, MEDLINE. She knows she needs to search more widely for her final assignment. For Alisha this is the first assignment of this nature and she is feeling a little overwhelmed so she and Charlotte decide to make an appointment with their subject librarian.

Scenario 3: Developing your healthcare/evidence-based practice dissertation

The students are learning to use the bibliographical databases to kick-start their search for appropriate literature to underpin their work. They have been given access to a complete sample dissertation (which is part of this book's electronic resource) which allows them to see first-hand how the architecture of a dissertation is constructed. All are conscious of how they must use their time wisely to ensure that they meet their deadlines.

Scenario 4: Preparing to use research evidence in your dissertation

At this point Sam is looking for qualitative studies to use in his dissertation and Sue is looking for randomised controlled trials that will help her answer her dissertation question. One of Sue's friends wants to examine historical literature. Alisha thinks she will need both qualitative and quantitative studies to support her topic and Charlotte is searching for systematic reviews and meta-analyses as well as randomised controlled trials.

Scenario 5: Critically appraising evidence

Having collected some relevant research articles, the students are faced with selecting appropriate critical appraisal tools to evaluate their selected papers. Sam has been advised to use Parahoo's critiquing approach, Sue and Charlotte find the Critical Appraisal Skills Programme (CASP) tools useful and Alisha also finds Greenhalgh's (2019) range of appraisal tools very helpful.

Scenario 6: Reflecting on your evidence-based dissertation/project/assignment journey

Just when Charlotte and Alisha thought they had completed the difficult parts of their assignments, they realised they still had to write a reflective element. They agreed it is easy to overlook the smaller components of the set work and to leave themselves little time for it. They have come to realise the importance of reflection and Charlotte discusses frameworks that might help get them started. Sue and Sam have a similar conversation and help each other to apply Gibbs' cycle of reflection to their work.

Section 1 **Starting your dissertation journey**

Sue is a senior staff nurse who works in an elderly care unit of a large tertiary teaching hospital. She entered nursing late after having a family and completed her enhanced diploma in adult nursing four years earlier. Her ward manager has sponsored her to undertake a 'top-up degree' programme at her local university. The programme she has enrolled on is specially designed to allow enhanced/advanced diplomate holders to progress towards gaining an honours degree classification to bring their academic qualifications up to the standard of initial nurse training today. In essence, the course entails attending a number of taught study days, where she will learn about the nuts and bolts of understanding evidence-based practice. The assessment, if successfully completed, will confer upon her a degree classification that is based on the submission of a 10 000-word dissertation. Sue has not opened a textbook for nearly five years and although she tries to keep up to date by reading a nursing journal which her ward subscribes to, she is full of trepidation about the course she has enrolled on.

Her good friend and neighbour, Sam, aged 31, works in the local children's hospital as a ward manager. He is already a graduate, having completed a degree in children's nursing some 10 years ago. Sam, likewise, has been out of the studying habit for many years. He is now seeking to become a clinical nurse specialist and has been fortunate to receive funding from his hospital to undertake an MSc in Nursing at the same university as Sue. Sam has a 'learning difference' and is dyslexic. The dissertation element of the MSc programme is similar to an undergraduate dissertation; it is in the form of a critical review of the evidence base for practice but this time is 20 000 words in length. Sam is equally worried about completing the dissertation element of the course.

Alisha left school without taking A-levels; she sought employment as a healthcare assistant at her local NHS Trust. Her ward managers recognised that Alisha had potential and when the new Nursing Associate Foundation Degree by the local university was launched in 2018 they sponsored her to undertake this new course. Alisha is now in her second and final year and is looking forward to registering with the Nursing and Midwifery Council as a qualified Nursing Associate. She must successfully complete an evidence-based practice project of 4000 words before completing the course. She and her friend Charlotte, who is a third-year student nurse, often meet in the library.

Charlotte is a third-year undergraduate student nurse and has been recently assessed as having a learning difference. She has been having regular support meetings with the faculty learning support manager. She has to write a 7000-word evidence-based practice assignment based on a topic of interest arising from her clinical placement experience.

Sue and Sam are facing the next challenge in their academic journey – the writing and completion of a dissertation. There is something about the dissertation that unsettles the two friends, which might be related to the size of the assignment or the freedom in choosing a project title. In reality, the dissertation gives them great freedom to choose what excites them as professionals working in clinical domains, but there are some principles that each will have to follow in developing their ideas. Charlotte and Alisha have been advised to reflect on their clinical experience to date to help them identify either gaps in their knowledge or occasions when they have become aware of different approaches to care for patients with similar conditions. They are reminded that the purpose of evidence-based practice is to ensure that clinical decisions are based on the best, most reliable evidence.

Chapter 1 **Starting the journey of your final-year project**

Megan Bonner-Janes
University of Southampton, UK

What is a final-year project?

The landscape of nurse training is evolving to become more flexible and accessible. Whether you have embarked on an apprenticeship leading to a degree in nursing or a foundation degree nursing associate qualification, are attending a higher education institution and undertaking a full-time direct entry degree in nursing, or perhaps you were awarded your nursing registration before the profession became all-graduate in 2013 and have now chosen to 'top-up' to a BSc or BN, you will be required to complete a final year project.

There are variations in the names awarded to these projects between education providers; dissertation, research project, evidenced-based practice project or portfolio for example. The form, structure and expected content of this project will also vary between institutions, with some requiring a 'traditional' 10 000-word evidence-based practice enquiry, while others may request a significantly shorter literature review, aimed at writing for a specific relevant journal with a view to publication. This might sound unfairly disparate, but often it is easier to work with a larger word count than it is a restricted one. Perhaps you will be required to critique the literature underpinning a specific piece of healthcare guidance, and then design an audit to test whether the recommendations are happening in practice.

Although there are many potential methodologies (research word for recipe) that you could be asked to follow, there are nevertheless commonalities between them all which remain constant, and so for the purposes of this book, we will refer to this polynymous piece of work as a 'final year project' or 'dissertation'.

This chapter is based on an earlier chapter by Sheila Reading.

How to Write Your Nursing Dissertation, Second Edition.
Edited by Alan Glasper and Diane Carpenter.
© 2021 John Wiley & Sons Ltd. Published 2021 by John Wiley & Sons Ltd.
Companion website: www.wiley.com/go/glasper/nursingdissertation2e

It is unlikely at undergraduate level that you would be asked to generate any new empirical evidence, meaning you will not be conducting research to generate new evidence yourself; rather you will be required to focus on a specific topic by systematically reviewing the literature in relation to that topic.

Other potential common features of a final-year project include:

- larger word count than other essays in the same programme;
- a requirement for you to show understanding of research methods and methodologies;
- a requirement for you to demonstrate your ability to be analytical and critical in your thinking and writing
- more credits than other essays (generally double the credit weighting compared with other assignments in the same programme).

A final-year project is often viewed as the culmination of a programme of learning which helps consolidate the student's knowledge, skills and understanding of the research base of the discipline.

Whether you are accessing a foundation degree to become a Nursing Associate, or are a fully registered nurse undertaking postgraduate study, it is essential to understand the task required of you.

Scenario

Alisha left school without taking A-levels; she sought employment as a healthcare assistant at her local NHS Trust. Her ward managers recognised that Alisha had potential and when the new Nursing Associate Foundation Degree by the local university was launched in 2018 they sponsored her to undertake this new course. Alisha is now in her second and final year and is looking forward to registering with the Nursing and Midwifery Council as a qualified Nursing Associate. However, Alisha must successfully complete an evidence-based practice project of 4000 words before completing the course. She and her friend Charlotte, who is a third-year student nurse, often meet in the library.

Charlotte is a third-year undergraduate student nurse and has been recently assessed as having a learning difference. She has been having regular support meetings with the faculty learning support manager. She has to write a 7000-word evidence-based practice assignment.

Sue, a senior staff nurse, has an Advanced Diploma in Nursing and is aware of the move to an all-graduate profession for new applicants to nursing. This has prompted her to embark on a 'top-up degree' programme at a nearby university to enable her to achieve graduate status. To meet the programme

requirements she will need to complete a 10 000-word evidence-based practice final-year project (dissertation).

Sam, a friend of Sue, is a ward manager and graduated with a Bachelor in
Nursing degree 10 years earlier and now wants to study for an MSc in
Nursing. For the MSc evidence-based practice final-year project he will have
to write a thesis of 20 000 words in length.

SUE: 'Why do we have to write such a long final year project?'

SAM: 'That is a good question Sue. We should first explore what an evi-
        dence-based practice final-year project is so we can understand why it
        is a significant aspect of our degree programmes and what we need to
        achieve. This article I have been reading indicates some key aspects of
        a final-year project.'

Activity 1.1

Before reading further it will be helpful for you to consider exactly what the
module requirements are for your final-year project. What is the task that you
have been set?

Talk to other people who have undertaken the task previously, or who are
currently undertaking the same project, to determine how they have
approached or intend to approach the task. It is likely that your course will
provide a number of exemplars of previous projects.

Note that the website that accompanies this book also has exemplar projects available, take a look to see which most closely resembles the project you
are undertaking.

Why do nurses need to do a research-based project?

The Nursing and Midwifery Council (NMC) is the regulatory body for registered nurses and nurses in training across England, Wales, Scotland and
Northern Ireland. They provide the standards of competence which underpin nursing practice and education. In *Future Nurse: Standards for Proficiency
for Registered Nurses* it states:

> The confidence and ability to think critically, apply knowledge and skills,
> and provide expert, evidence-based, direct nursing care therefore lies at
> the centre of all registered nursing practice.

(NMC 2018:3)

Healthcare practitioners need to be able to ask questions about practice, access healthcare research and evidence, and report the key ideas and findings effectively and accurately to others. Preparing a final-year project will provide you with the skills that you need to be able to search for, and critically evaluate, relevant theoretical knowledge and literature, which will underpin your practice, improve your knowledge, inform your practice, and therefore improve outcomes for patients and service users.

It is therefore the process of writing a final-year project that is arguably more important than the final project document itself. Production of a final-year evidence-based project is the primary means to achieving an honours or a master's degree.

Undergraduate versus postgraduate projects

Normally an undergraduate project will be based on a critique of a small selection of evidence and be applied to one focused aspect of practice. It will provide insight and hands-on experience of the process of engaging in evidence-based practice and should inform individual or local professional clinical practice.

The requirement of a master's programme is that the evidence-based project demonstrates how the student has 'mastered' a core aspect of healthcare practice, related research knowledge and discipline-related content.

There is a *qualitative* difference between the master's final-year project and the undergraduate final-year project as well as the *quantitative* difference recognised by the word allowance. This normally relates to the depth, breadth and analysis demonstrated in the written work. A master's final-year project will systematically critique a greater amount of evidence from a range of different sources, demonstrating a significant appreciation of underlying issues, application, and impact of the findings for the wider practice context.

Undergraduate evidence-based practice projects tend to focus on 'what' and 'where' questions related to practice, while master's level work will move on to asking more analytical questions that focus on the 'how' and 'why' of practice.

The UK Quality Assurance Agency (QAA) Subject Benchmark Statement provides a means of describing standards for the award of qualifications at a given level. The capabilities and attributes of those who undertake final-year projects for particular qualifications should demonstrate the appropriate level of study. This is always indicated in the programme final-year project assignment guidelines and the learning outcomes made available to students. More detail on this can be found in Chapter 2.

What are the features of a degree education?

Increasingly, degree programmes and foundation degree nursing associate courses are aligned with the achievement of defined 'graduate attributes'. Many higher education institutions have identified their own specific graduate attributes. These usually focus on skills which are valuable for, and transferable to, work-based contexts. Graduate attributes support learners in meeting the needs of a complex, challenging and constantly changing environment of employment. They include more than just the academic or professional skills of the discipline and demonstrate skills needed to be independent, autonomous and lifelong learners, which are viewed as important characteristics of being a graduate. Graduate attributes include personal qualities, skills and knowledge gained as a result of engaging in study. They include qualities such as adopting academic approaches to thinking which demonstrate openness to new ways of responding to unfamiliar situations and challenges with intellectual curiosity.

In addition to developing skills in information retrieval and critiquing research evidence, completing a degree or foundation degree equips individuals with highly prized transferable skills such as problem solving, project management and report writing that can significantly enhance professional communication and practice. In a study to elucidate research-related graduate attributes, Laidlaw *et al.* (2009) found evidence to support the case for final-year projects helping achieve both clinical and research-related graduate attributes for medical undergraduates. The attributes included an inquiring mind, core knowledge, critical appraisal, understanding the evidence base for professional practice, understanding ethics and governance, and an ability to communicate. Each of these graduate attributes could be argued as being relevant for other healthcare professionals.

Completing a foundation degree and/or subsequently an honours degree is often a precursor to further academic study such as a postgraduate masters or doctoral studies. A master's final-year project will build on previous knowledge gained at undergraduate level and develop new understandings

---

Tip

As well as significant differences in word length and the scope and depth of analysis required, the period of time available to complete and the expected hours of self-directed study differ between an undergraduate and postgraduate masters final-year project. Make sure you have explored in detail the final-year project requirements of your programme and use them to help you organise and plan for the task ahead.

and a greater breadth and depth of learning. Each stage is part of a progressive development of research knowledge and skills. This may be part of developing a clinical academic career pathway that integrates research and education to improve the use of research, and other evidence, in clinical practice (UKCRC, 2007).

Activity 1.2

Think about all the reasons why you want to become a nursing associate or registered nurse, and the reasons for choosing to study at the level you are. Prioritise the items and write a short summary statement to refer back to later.

Features of a final-year project

A final-year project is an extended and substantial piece of work carried out independently. It is common to have a link with a group of peers who are also completing a final-year project with the same submission date and to have a link with a member of the university staff who will supervise and offer academic support. The final-year project is quite different from other assignments in terms of its depth and the length of time engaged with it. While it may be divided into sections or chapters, it needs to demonstrate a coherent and well-structured format that poses a question which is then addressed and answered in relation to a specific practice issue.

The initial choice of topic selected can increase the personal and professional depth of understanding on the subject. Very often the breadth of knowledge may be extended into unexpected areas. For example, a recent final-year project which focused on enhancing the care of people with long-term conditions in one NHS Trust led the student to an exploration of concepts of clinical leadership, while another student, also focusing on long-term conditions, explored the evidence for promoting approaches to self-care.

Whatever topic is chosen, it is important to remember that sustained motivation to undertake a final-year project requires considerable enthusiasm for both the subject and the process, over an extended period of time.

The key features of a final-year project may include:

- Title
- Well-framed question
- Clear aims and objectives
- Search strategy for best evidence
- Critical appraisal of research or other best evidence
- Discussion of results and implication for practice.

Discussion point

If you have been seconded or are being funded by an employer, you might find that they allocate you a topic for your project, usually because it is specific to, and enhances practice in, your particular practice area.

You may consider this to be helpful, because it limits what can feel like an overwhelming choice of inquiries . . . *but* . . . remember that it is important to choose a subject which inspires you, because you are the one who has to 'live and breathe' it for the duration. If you find yourself bored with reading around the subject after the initial literature search, this might not be the topic for you!

Have a think about what really captures your interest, and then discuss with your manager how much wiggle room there is for negotiation of topic. It might be that your personal choice is related to your practice, which will assist the negotiation, but remember that the process of learning how to search for and critically assess literature is what will enhance your practice, not the findings of the project itself necessarily.

All these aspects will be covered and discussed in the various chapters of this book.

Additionally, this will all have to be written up in a readable style, communicating the relevant information and presented in an understandable format according to regulations, and submitted on time. Penalties for breaching guidance and regulations may be applied.

Producing a final-year project demonstrates and communicates that you have consolidated a range of skills including, intellectual, professional, information-seeking, critical analysis and synthesis of knowledge.

Planning your final-year project: essential considerations

Chapter 2 gives further details on how final-year projects are planned.

Planning your available time

Some students find the use of Gantt charts (Table 1.1) helpful. It is important to be clear about how much time to allocate to each step of the process. Several stages may be undertaken at a time and undertaking a final-year project is not always a linear process.

It is sensible to remember that things do not always run according to plan. Life events can interfere and mean that work is delayed. It makes sense to build in time for some slippage to prevent last minute panic in meeting the

Table 1.1   Example of a Gantt chart.

	Oct	Nov	Dec	Jan	Feb	Mar	April	May	June
Select topic	———→								
Search and select evidence	———————————→							
Critically appraise evidence			———————————→					
Write up chapters	——————————————————————————→							
Conclusions/ discussion					——————————————→			

deadline for submission. Do allow time for making final revisions and checking for spelling or other errors.

**Begin writing early: produce drafts to show others and get
feedback**
While the list of things to do indicated above gives an outline of the structure
for a typical written final-year project, careful thought is needed about how
best to present the final coherent project.

Reading other final-year projects written by students who have completed
similar programmes is always a good resource for considering how to frame
your headings, sections and chapters. However, each final-year project is
unique, and support from a personal tutor in interpreting the assignment
guidelines to apply to your own project is always essential.

At times it can be difficult to be certain where, for example, the writing on
the results section should end and when the conclusions begin. It is important to weave all the sections together into the whole which is the final written project.

It is important to avoid writing too descriptively. Remember you need to
adopt an academic approach, demonstrating your ability to think critically
and analytically and to synthesise conclusions from all the information you
have gathered.

Get support from others
Enlist family and friends to encourage you in keeping on task, and work with
peers on the programme who are going through the same experience as you.
Email them, set up group discussions on messaging apps, or meet informally

to discuss aspects of each other's work and for mutual support. It is a common phenomenon to get 'too close' to your own work to see the flaws or how to resolve them. It is generally easier to be objective about someone else's work. For this reason, supporting other students with the difficulties they are encountering with their work can be of benefit to your own work.

Take opportunities offered to present your ideas to the programme group or your personal tutor in order to get supportive feedback. Some universities have special sections of their electronic learning platforms (e.g. Backboard or Microsoft Teams) which feature student chat-rooms where information can be exchanged.

Adopt the help of 'critical readers'. It might sound counterintuitive, but sometimes the best people to proofread work are not necessarily those who are familiar with your topic, or even with healthcare. This is because someone with understanding of the subject can subconsciously fill in gaps in knowledge, whereas someone with no knowledge will require clarification if the writing is not clear enough.

Your proofreader will need to be honest with you and receiving feedback is hard, so try not to get defensive or they might not help again in the future! As well as content, they need to comment on whether the work is coherent and well structured. You might feel that comments relating to SPaG (spelling, punctuation and grammar) by your reader is being picky, but these things can impact the meaning of a sentence, which could make you look like you lack understanding – so better that they spot the errors before your marker does.

Finally, back up everything you save on your computer.

Tip

- Buy several (minimum four megabytes) data/memory sticks/USB flash drives to store copies of your work.
- Create a folder entitled 'My final year project' with sub-folders for each individual chapter.

Completing your final-year project and gaining a good classification

Because the final-year project at foundation degree/undergraduate or postgraduate level makes a significant contribution in terms of credits gained and to the student's final classification, it is often an important priority for students to gain a good result.

Make sure you meet the deadlines for submitting the final-year project for marking and that you are not rushed towards the end. Being short of time can lead to you having to take shortcuts and potentially reduce the time available to complete your writing to the required standard. Remember time is needed to refine drafts, ensure accurate reference lists, and check for typographical and other errors related to the general presentation before the final year project is submitted. In some institutions they will expect you to have your project bound, which can take at least one week, so this will need to be factored in. Be clear about the written style (font and spacing) and final presentation format required by your university and foundation degree/honours degree/MSc programme.

To achieve a good grade you will need to look at the module assignment guidelines and learning outcomes and the marking criteria (Table 1.2). Universities normally explain the basis on which student final-year projects are assessed in order to guide student learning and, importantly, to ensure work is marked fairly and consistently. It is very important that as a student you are familiar with the final-year project requirements and marking guidance. Often a module handbook is produced by the university that will give details of the final-year project expectations and the explicit marking criteria by which they will be assessed. This can be discussed with your personal tutor at an early stage and as you complete written sections or chapters. Part of your own learning is to develop your skills in self-assessment so you can recognise the standard of work which you are capable of and need to aim for in order to ensure the desired grade.

Table 1.2 Example of possible evidence-based final-year project marking criteria.

Category	Relative importance (%)
Presentation (structure, language, referencing)	8
Abstract (accuracy, relevance and clarity	2
Introduction (background to project, issues to be addressed, background reading, framing of the question)	20
Identification and selection of best evidence (retrieval of evidence, search strategy and terms, rationale for criteria to select or reject evidence, audit trail)	20
Critical appraisal of evidence (rationale for selection of critiquing framework/tool, judgement of evidence, rigour, addresses the question, research understanding)	25
Conclusions and implications for practice (conclusions well drawn from selected evidence, skills of analysis and evaluation, relevance to practice, application to practice)	15
Discussion and plan for implementation	10

Chapter 1

Don't panic!

It is entirely understandable and quite usual to feel overwhelmed or anxious about such an undertaking, but with more than 650 000 qualified nurses working in the UK currently (Office of National Statistics, 2020) there is plenty of evidence that this is an entirely achievable and rewarding endeavour. You are not alone, link in with fellow students past and current, keep talking to your personal tutor and any work colleagues who have done the same or similar.

Be organised and systematic in your approach, and don't become an ostrich – if any personal or health issues are impacting on your study, or you get a study block, talk to your tutor as soon as possible, as they can provide advice and support (more on getting the most from your tutor/supervisor can be found in Chapter 12).

Activity 1.3

Find out about different learning/study styles and what works for you. Perhaps you work best first thing in the morning or last thing at night? Are you a 'little and often' person or a last-minute crammer? Perhaps you have carer responsibilities which will put restrictions on the time you have to study?

Take some time to think about all of the things that will impact on your study, whether positive or negative, and take some time to consider how you will manage them, or use them to your advantage.

There are plenty of study skills books online or in the library which offer practical advice on maintaining well-being while studying.

References

Laidlaw, A., Guild, S. & Struthers, J. (2009) Graduate attributes in the disciplines of medicine, dentistry and veterinary medicine: a survey of expert opinions. *BioMed Central Medical Education*, **9**, 28.

NMC (2018) *Future Nurse: Standards for Proficiency for Registered Nurses.* Nursing and Midwifery Council, London.

Office of National Statistics (2020) Annual number of nurses in the United Kingdom (UK) from 2010 to 2019. https://www.statista.com/statistics/318922/number-of-nurses-in-the-uk/

UKCRC Subcommittee for Nurses in Clinical Research (2007) *Developing the best research professionals. Qualified graduate nurses: recommendations for preparing and supporting clinical academic nurses of the future.* UK Clinical Research Collaboration. Available at https://www.ukcrc.org/reports/

For further resources for this chapter visit the companion website at
 www.wiley.com/go/glasper/nursingdissertation2e

Chapter 2 Introduction to writing your evidence-based practice dissertation/project

Alan Glasper[1], and Diane Carpenter[2]
[1]*University of Southampton, UK*
[2]*University of Plymouth, UK*

Scenario

Sue, Alisha, Charlotte and Sam are facing the next challenge in their academic journey – the writing and completion of a dissertation/project or evidence-informed decision-making project/assignment. There is something about the dissertation/project/assignment that unsettles the four students, which might be related to the size of the assignment or the freedom in choosing a project title. In reality, the project gives them great freedom to choose what excites them as healthcare workers working in clinical domains, but there are some principles that each will have to follow in developing their ideas.

Most healthcare students undertaking an undergraduate or postgraduate course have to submit a dissertation/project/assignment as part of the assessment process. The learning outcomes of these may differ but the basic architecture remains the same.

Sample guidelines for students undertaking a nursing associate project, an undergraduate healthcare project/dissertation or a master's degree project

All students need to read carefully the particular university assessment guidelines for whichever course they are undertaking. Dissertations/projects or evidence-based assignments usually take the form of an evidence-based practice

This chapter is based on an earlier chapter by Alan Glasper and Colin Rees

---

How to Write Your Nursing Dissertation, Second Edition.
Edited by Alan Glasper and Diane Carpenter.
© 2021 John Wiley & Sons Ltd. Published 2021 by John Wiley & Sons Ltd.
Companion website: www.wiley.com/go/glasper/nursingdissertation2e

project that focuses in depth on a clinical/practice focused issue. Students normally identify an issue arising from their own practice area, and will further develop this into a question to guide the dissertation/project/assignment.

Typical dissertations/projects/assignments will include some or all of the following sections.

- Introduction and rationale for selection of the topic area.
- Review of literature relating to the subject area leading to the generation of the research question or recommendations for practice.
- Strategy for collection of evidence, including database search range/terminology.
- Critical appraisal and evaluation of evidence relating to the topic.
- Analysis of the findings.
- Discussion and synthesis of the extent to which the evidence reviewed answers the research question.
- Critical discussion on the potential implementation of the project findings to practice, via clinical audit incorporating consideration of the culture of the organisation, leadership styles and new management strategies best suited to achieve this.

Typical learning outcomes for a nursing associate course 2000-word literature review

At the point of registration, the nursing associate will be able to, among other things, describe the principles of research and how research findings are used to inform evidence-based practice, as follows.

1. Develop knowledge and understanding regarding the research process, which underpins contemporary evidence-based practice.
2. Demonstrate an ability to undertake a review of the literature using a variety of search methods.
3. Show an understanding of how literature can be appraised.
4. Appreciate the use of the clinical audit process as a way of measuring current provision of care.
5. Demonstrate the skills to further develop and innovate service delivery to patients in order to improve and promote the delivery of high-quality, safe and effective care.

Typical learning outcomes for an undergraduate evidence-based practice dissertation/project

1. Demonstrate the ability to systematically search and critically appraise evidence, including literature/primary research/systematic

    reviews/clinical guidelines using an appropriate critical appraisal framework(s).

2. Critically analyse practice and identify a clinical issue for exploration.
3. Demonstrate a critical awareness and knowledge of research methodology.
4. Reflect on the breadth of evidence that underpins practice.
5. Derive solutions to problems based on the collection, interrogation and interpretation of information and data obtained from a variety of sources, and draw on established analytical techniques in the broad field of health and social care.
6. Demonstrate self-reflection and an understanding of the limitations of the key concepts of the underpinning disciplines.
7. Demonstrate confidence in understanding, manipulating, interpreting and presenting numerical narrative data.
8. Demonstrate an understanding of the role of the student and supervisor.
9. Identify a question for an evidence-based practice project to inform a proposal and dissertation/project.
10. Consider ways in which styles of leadership and organisational culture impact on effective care delivery within a range of practice arenas.
11. Critically discuss the barriers and behaviours which may undermine the achievement of excellent practice.
12. Critically appraise the barriers and opportunities that will impinge on evidence-based practice within clinical care, management, education and research.
13. Consider ways in which barriers to evidence-based practice could be reduced.
14. Critically evaluate the process by which evidence can be disseminated.
15. Gather and evaluate evidence and information from a wide range of sources: to think logically, systematically and conceptually; to draw reasoned conclusions or to reach sustainable judgements, and to apply these to practice.

Typical learning outcomes for a postgraduate evidence-based practice dissertation/project

1. Demonstrate initiative, originality and justification for the construction of an original question/focus relevant to your practice/workplace, and within the wider context of health and social care.
2. Conduct an effective systematic search in relation to the question/focus that has been developed and critically appraise and evaluate the identified literature.

3. Demonstrate a comprehensive knowledge based on the different types of evidence, the research paradigms and approaches, and the ability to critically evaluate their relevance and contribution to your health and social care setting.
4. Critically analyse the relevance of any ethical and/or governance implications that may arise during the course of your enquiry.
5. Synthesise the evidence to address the original questions/focus and any associated issues significant to the chosen topic.
6. Demonstrate initiative in interpretation of the findings taking into account limitations and challenges of the implementation of evidence-based practice.
7. Justify the conclusions and recommendations based on insightful, comprehensive, realistic and well-reasoned arguments.
8. Demonstrate an extensive knowledge of a range of concepts and current research or professional issues in the chosen area of enquiry and demonstrate the ability to illustrate your unique project decision trail through the production of a coherent, logical, reflective and comprehensive report of the process, outcomes and implications of your enquiry.
9. Synthesise an innovative dissemination strategy to best influence evidence-based practice in your speciality.
10. Critically reflect on your project activity and learning and its contribution to your future practice/role.

The dissertation/project/assignment

For many students, the idea of producing a 10 000 (undergraduate) word or 20 000 (postgraduate master's course) word dissertation/project is a daunting one, despite this rising to 80 000 words for a PhD.

However, it need not be overwhelming. This chapter has been designed to help you understand what is required as you embark on this personal academic journey. It is important to set yourself achievable and manageable target dates for each stage of your dissertation/project journey (and try to keep to them!). Many universities will allocate you an educational supervisor who will guide and support you through the process.

Selecting a topic area

Many of you will have an idea of the topic you wish to explore in your dissertation/project and will pose or frame an evidence-based question usually related to your own sphere of practice. Once you have framed a question, you will search the scholarly literature for evidence to allow you to answer your question. This will be achieved through a comprehensive process we describe in this book involving a range of reputable databases. Normally you can trust your own university or hospital librarian to help you with this task. Some universities will ask you to submit a written proposal prior to the commencement of your dissertation/project. This may be formative (no grade allocated) or summative (where a mark is given and this contributes to the total mark awarded for the dissertation/project). The proposal will require a comprehensive outline of the proposed evidence-based practice project and will provide the opportunity for feedback and consideration prior to commencing the dissertation/project.

Supervision

Most universities have a code of conduct relating to supervision (where provided) and it is normally the responsibility of the student to consult their supervisor to discuss any problems and to seek guidance on aspects of the work. The amount of supervision time students are entitled to also varies depending on the level of the course being undertaken, with more for a PhD and less for an undergraduate or nursing associate course.

Educational supervision will usually be provided by a member of the academic team who has experience either in the area of the student's project or of the methodology to be used. A supervisor should meet the following criteria:

- evidence of previous research work and experience;
- ideally have an appropriate background in the area of the project or the methodology used in the student's project.

Submission deadline

It is the student's responsibility to complete and submit the dissertation/project by the deadline stipulated by the individual university. This is usually an academic semester. All students in university settings will have access to processes to request mitigation or special consideration. All students should read the relevant policy in their own university student handbook.

Guidelines for students undertaking a nursing associate evidence-based practice assignment

These projects will vary from university to university but the schedule below is a guideline for a 2000-word evidence-based literature review assignment. Suggested word limits for each section are approximate.

- Title page (outlining the relevant module code, your student number, the date of submission and the title of your essay).

- Introduction: selecting and justifying a clinical issue and formulation of topic question (250 words).
- Main body:
  - Identification of search terms and justification for appropriate sources of evidence (150 words).
  - Literature search strategy (200 words with diagrammatic illustration, e.g. PRISMA flow diagram) resulting in selection of two to four research articles.
  - Discussion of articles including some critical comment (750 words).
  - Synthesis of findings (250 words).
  - Application or relevance to practice (200 words).
- Conclusion (200 words).
- Reference list.

Guidelines for students undertaking an undergraduate evidence-based practice final project

These projects will vary from university to university but the schedule described here is typical of a final evidence-based assignment.

The summative 7000-word written report of the project will be structured in chapters (as indicated in the following list) and will demonstrate your ability to develop a plan to improve an aspect of professional practice. This will include identifying and justifying a clinical issue, critically appraising clinical guideline recommendations that address this issue, designing a clinical audit aiming to improve practice to reflect guideline recommendations, and exploring the leadership implications of engaging other practitioners in the improvement project.

The following sections should be included:

- Title page (outlining the relevant module code, your student number, the date of submission and the title of your essay)
- Contents page
- List of tables (if applicable)
- List of figures (if applicable)
- Glossary
- Acknowledgements
- Chapter 1: Selecting and justifying a clinical issue
- Chapter 2: Identifying and appraising a clinical guideline
- Chapter 3: Audit proposal
- Chapter 4: Implementation and change
- Reference list.

Guidelines for students undertaking an undergraduate evidence-based practice dissertation

Although these will vary from university to university, the schedule described here is typical.

- Students are required to submit a dissertation/project of up to 10 000 words, excluding diagrams, appendices, references and bibliography.
- The dissertation/project must be submitted electronically according to the university's criteria.
- Typical dissertation/projects are usually set out as follows:
  - Title page containing:
    Name of university, year and faculty or school
    Full name and number of student
    Title of course
    Title of the dissertation/project
    Word count.
  - Contents page listing:
    Abstract
    Acknowledgements
    Introduction
    Literature review
    Method
    Results
    Discussion of results
    Conclusions and recommendations for practice
    References (using the modified Harvard system)
    List of tables/figures
    Glossary of terms or abbreviations
    Appendices.
- All pages must be numbered centrally at the foot of each page.
- Presentation is important: poor or hurried proofreading will affect the quality of the dissertation/project. Remember to use grammar and spell-check.
- A signed statement of originality and authorship is usually required; this may include the word count for the work. Usually, everything before the first page of the introduction is not included in the word count; the references and appendices are, similarly, not included in the word count, but do check for local variations. You will be guided locally as to where this statement sheet should be placed and if it is required to be 'bound' into the dissertation/project. Most dissertations are now required to be submitted online, but must still conform to the recognised layout.

A frequent concern is how long each section should be. This is not easy to answer, as it will depend on available information for the sections and what is required in your educational institution. However, Table 2.1 gives some indication of typical sections and approximate word counts.

Chapter 2

Table 2.1 Sections, their purpose and approximate word counts (master's level) for healthcare dissertation/project.

Section title	Reason for inclusion	Approximate word count	Evidence-based process
Abstract	Provide a succinct summary of dissertation/project. Usually written as a one single-spaced paragraph	300–500	
Introduction/ Background	Orientates the reader to the practice-focused issue: states origin of the study (personal/ professional influences); why the area invites investigation. The question is presented clarifying the explicit link to the identified clinical area of enquiry	1500–2000	Generating the evidence
Selection and identification of the evidence	Presents the search strategy and database, including the search terms used, to illustrate depth and breadth of search. Clarifies rationale for choice of criteria used to select and reject evidence for critical appraisal	1500–2000	Selecting the evidence
Critical appraisal of selected evidence	Identifies evidence that is relevant to the practice-related question and critically appraises this evidence through the use of a critiquing tool. Applies the selected evidence to the question set	3000	Appraising the evidence
Conclusion and implications	Offers conclusions which address the question and which are drawn from the presented argument. Reviews how far the evidence answers the question	1500	Determining the worth of the evidence
Plan for implementation	Offers an outline plan for implementation and dissemination. Critical discussion should demonstrate consideration of influencing factors such as the culture of the organisation, leadership styles and change management strategies best suited to achieve the plan	1500	Implementing the evidence

Guidelines for a typical postgraduate evidence-based practice dissertation/project module learning outcomes

The structure of postgraduate evidence-based practice dissertation/projects can vary and you should follow any guidelines you are given. However, Table 2.2 provides a typical outline.

Table 2.2 Guideline for sections within the dissertation/project.

Section	Guideline
Title page	This should detail the university, school, award, candidate's name and dissertation/project title (not included in the word count)
Abstract	This should be a concise and precise summary of the entire dissertation/project. It is usually presented as one single-spaced paragraph. A structured abstract is recommended but should be appropriate to the nature of the project (not included in the word count)
Acknowledgements	This page is optional (not included in the word count)
Contents	This should be detailed and accurate, covering all chapters, tables, figure and appendices (not included in the word count)
Chapter 1: Introduction	This should provide comprehensive information on the topic, the rationale for its selection, its context in terms of your practice and the wider agenda for evidence-based practice in health and social care. Arising from this introduction should come the development of the aim, often in the form of the original research or practice question(s)
Chapter 2: Literature review	This chapter details the systematic literature search strategy for the generation of data/evidence together with details of methods of appraisal. This may include any refining of the question(s), the results of the search activity and the selection of the key papers. There should be a clear decision-making trail through this chapter. It may be separate from or integrated within the following main section of the literature review chapter
Chapter 3: Critical appraisal and synthesis of data/evidence	This chapter should demonstrate an advanced ability to critically appraise and synthesise the evidence. An excellent knowledge of the relevant research paradigms, approaches and methods that are appropriate to the selected evidence and the topic should be presented. It is expected that you will be able to critically discuss the paradigms/approaches and offer a balanced exploration of the relative merits of each to practice and the selected topic. Ethical issues must be considered appropriately. There should be a thematic and integrated approach throughout, with clear practice/professional awareness. There should be a clear decision-making trail through this chapter leading to judgements on the quality of the evidence and hence what evidence can be discussed in relation to promoting evidence-based practice

(Continued)

Table 2.2   (Continued)

Section	Guideline
Chapter 4: Discussion (analysis of findings in context of wider literature and practice)	In addition to a discussion of findings in relation to the research/practice question(s), there should be original and creative recommendations for changing practice. Take into consideration the context of the practice setting, the current national and local health and social care agenda as well as the philosophy of evidence-based practice. You should explore where further development is needed to achieve evidence-based practice
Chapter 5: Dissemination strategy	The dissemination strategy will need to identify an extensive range of approaches, justified with relevant theory, for presenting a clear message and to communicate effectively your evidence-based results in order to make a contribution to your field of practice and to the development of the knowledge base of your discipline/practice
Chapter 6: Project analysis and conclusions	Critically review the methodology you used in the project, reflecting on learning achieved and continuing. The presentation of an overview of the project with clear conclusion
References	These must conform to your university's referencing presentation style; be accurate and complete in both the text and the reference list
Appendices	These should only provide additional evidence; the main body of work should be complete without them (these do not contribute to the word count)

Conclusion

Just like you, Sue, Charlotte, Alisha and Sam are facing the next challenge in their academic journey – the completion of the dissertation/project or evidence-based assignment. The remainder of this book explores some essential principles that each of you will have to follow in developing your ideas and in completing the evidence-based practice dissertation/project.

For further resources for this chapter visit the companion website at
www.wiley.com/go/glasper/nursingdissertation2e

Chapter 3 Clinical effectiveness and evidence-based practice: background and history

Mary O'Toole[1] and Alan Glasper[2]
[1]University of Plymouth, UK
[2]University of Southampton, UK

Scenario

Sue has attended the first class of her dissertation module that provides the background to evidence-based practice (EBP) and evidence-informed decision making (EIDM). She and Sam have got together with their laptops to trace for themselves the origins of EBP and EIDM. The clinical environments in which they (and you!) work now expect all staff to understand not only how to access up-to-date publications pertinent to changes in clinical practice, but also to understand the process through which new evidence is generated. Sue and Sam are trying to discover why the system is so important and how it all began. Charlotte and Alisha have recently attended a lecture on the origins and history of EBP.

Introduction

Although evidence-based practice (EBP) seems to have been part of healthcare culture for some time, it is in fact a relatively recent phenomenon. As it will underpin so much of what we cover in this book, we start this chapter with a brief background to EBP and its development. Sackett, Rosenberg and Haynes were among the early protagonists of the EBP movement (Bick and Graham, 2010) and their definition (Sackett *et al.*, 1997:2),

This chapter is based on an earlier chapter by Alan Glasper and Colin Rees

---

How to Write Your Nursing Dissertation, Second Edition.
Edited by Alan Glasper and Diane Carpenter.
© 2021 John Wiley & Sons Ltd. Published 2021 by John Wiley & Sons Ltd.
Companion website: www.wiley.com/go/glasper/nursingdissertation2e

> *. . . the conscientious, explicit and judicious use of current best evidence about the care of individual patients*

is still widely accepted by healthcare professionals. More recently, the term 'evidence-informed decision making' (EIDM) has become more widely used and is defined by the National Collaborating Centre for Methods and Tools as 'the process of distilling and disseminating the best available evidence from research, practice and experience and using that evidence to inform and improve public health policy and practice' (www.nccmt.ca/about/eiph)

A fundamental function of the Nursing and Midwifery Council (NMC) is to protect the public and a key professional standard is to 'Always practise in line with the best available evidence' (Standard 6; Nursing and Midwifery Council, 2018). The connection between these two ideals of protecting the public and the process of EBP has been outlined by a number of authors (Fineout-Overholt *et al.*, 2005; Parahoo, 2014). More recently, the National Institute for Health Research has published a Clinical Research Nurse Strategy (2019) stating that clinical research nurses, midwives and specialist community public health nurses have a vital role in the delivery of quality clinically researched care. A further important ingredient within EBP is a 'spirit of inquiry', described by Melnyk *et al.* (2009) as an 'ongoing curiosity about the best evidence to guide clinical decision making' and importantly a working culture that supports it.

The work of Fineout-Overholt *et al.* (2005) includes a step-by-step approach using a problem-solving approach to EBP that embodies Sackett's original principles. Additionally, the National Collaborating Centre for Methods and Tools details a model for EIDM (this is explored further at the end of the chapter).

Historical aspects of evidence-based practice

Ancient civilisations undoubtedly attempted to base their medical practice on the best evidence available at the time. Interestingly, Reid (2008) suggests that the first controlled trial is cited in the Bible in the Book of Daniel. Here, chapter 1, verses 1–21 clearly describe the comparison between two groups of children: one group were given the royal food, namely the meat and wine of King Nebuchadnezzar, and the second comparison group of children received a vegetarian diet in the form of pulses and drank only water. The aim of this comparative trial was to establish differences in 'countenance', which usually refers to appearance, especially of the face, and how it is perceived by others.

During this first biblical trial an unknown number of non-royal Israeli children and some of royal birth who were blemish free, wise, able to learn a language and with an understanding of science were given the food and drink of the conquering Persian king whose aim, presumably, was to eradicate dissent against the invaders by making some of these children part of his own royal court. Importantly, the gender mix of these groups was not stated.

The story unfolds that the boy Daniel and three other royal Israeli children, presumably to avoid breaking kosher laws, requested permission from the king's officer, the prince of the eunuchs, 'not to defile himself' with the 'daily rations from the king's food and from the wine he drank' (Kaptchuk and Kerr, 2004). According to the Bible, the prince of the eunuchs was very fond of Daniel, who was able to persuade him to undertake what was in effect a 10-day prospective comparative study. Daniel's group of four boys ate pulses (beans) and drank water and the remainder ate the king's food. After the 10 days, Daniel and the three other Israeli royal boys of royal blood had a better countenance than the other Israeli children who enjoyed the diet of the king.

Although this first trial is frequently referred to within the annals of EBP, Stolberg *et al.* (2004) have some concerns about it, not least the lack of science in the randomisation of the individuals participating in the trial. This is important as, without it, there could have been biasing factors (i.e. characteristics that might distort the results) in the physical make-up of the two groups and this might have influenced the outcome rather than the type of food. The other major problem you might have considered is the lack of a measure of 'countenance' and how comparisons could have objectively been made between the two groups.

History has also provided other examples of attempts to produce 'evidence' to answer clinical questions. Harvie (2002) describes how Lind, a young naval surgeon's assistant, conducted the first controlled clinical trial in the quest to discover the cause of scurvy, a condition caused by nutritional deficiency that killed many sailors and passengers on long voyages in the 1700s. In 1747, Lind conducted a trial on 12 men with scurvy where one group ($n = 2$) received two oranges and one lemon a day. These two men made a good recovery, whereas the others who were given non-citrus treatments, including sea water, consequently did not recover. Despite the evidence, it was to be another 48 years before the British Admiralty began to issue lemon juice to naval seamen for the prevention of scurvy (Box 3.1).

> **Box 3.1   Why the English are called Limeys**
> It would have been logical to have nicknamed the English 'Lemonies' after their conquest of scurvy. However, by the mid-nineteenth century the British government decided to spend its resources on West Indian limes rather than Mediterranean lemons, believing that limes were very similar to lemons. Tragically, the amount of vitamin C in limes is significantly less than in lemons, and scurvy returned to blight the British Royal Navy. Although the North Americans still refer to the British as Limeys, had a true randomised controlled trial been conducted, they would in all probability now be called 'Rosies'.
>   Why? The answer is that rose hips contain vast amounts of vitamin C and are freely available in the British countryside!

Chapter 3

The contribution of the nursing profession to evidence-based practice

Within nursing, the use of data as a source of decision making can be traced back to Florence Nightingale (McDonald, 2001) who powerfully demonstrated her commitment to systematic data collection. After her return from the Crimean war, Nightingale was haunted by the excessive loss of life, where disease caused more deaths than bullets by a factor of seven. She began to lobby for a real investigation into the root cause of this and began to analyse and present data in a way that even a non-statistician could understand. Her work was illustrated with the use of diagrams and Nightingale is credited with the development of colour-coded bar charts and pie charts to illustrate her findings on the death rates of soldiers from infection. Her ability to be ahead of her time is also illustrated by her use of this approach to data collection and presentation to highlight the benefits of a trained nursing workforce compared to that of an untrained workforce (McDonald, 2001).

The 1944 patulin (a derivative of penicillin) trial for the treatment of the common cold and the 1948 streptomycin trial for tuberculosis were both designed with true randomisation and controls in place (Kaptchuk and Kerr, 2004). The era of modern EBP was about to begin.

How is evidence sourced?

EBP is a thoughtful integration of the best available evidence coupled with clinical expertise and the patient's wishes. What is also important and sometimes forgotten is the lived experience of the patient. In their Clinical Research Nurse Strategy, the National Institute for Health Research (2019) advocate for a clinical research culture that is patient and public focused. The strategy advises actively promoting patient involvement and engagement throughout the research pathway, including priority setting (www.nihr.ac.uk).

Healthcare practitioners should aim to address healthcare questions with an evaluative and quantitative approach. EBP allows the practitioner to assess current and past research, clinical guidelines and other information resources to identify relevant literature, while differentiating between high-quality and low-quality findings.

Melnyk *et al.* (2010) identify six fundamental steps in EBP.

- *Step 1: Formulate a question.* This can be achieved using the PICO or similar format (outlined in Chapter 9).
- *Step 2: Find the evidence.* Interrogate research databases such as MEDLINE, CINAHL, Cochrane, Joanna Briggs and so on, not forgetting grey literature (see Chapters 6 and 7 which cover this in detail).
- *Step 3: Appraise the evidence.* Use one of the many critiquing tools available to undertake critical appraisal. This book will concentrate on only a small number of tools. However, Melnyk *et al.* (2010) advise nurses who are busy to initially use what they call Rapid Critical Appraisal, which uses three key questions to allow a quick evaluation of what a particular paper offers:
  - ○ Are the results of the study valid?
  - ○ What are the results and are they important?
  - ○ Will the results help me care for my patients?
- *Step 4: Integrate the evidence.* This should be combined with clinical expertise and patient preferences and values in applying the evidence. After the studies have been critiqued, the next step is to determine the value of the evidence by synthesising their combined weight to check if they all come to a similar conclusion that will warrant a change in clinical practice. Unfortunately, making changes in practice is not a simple process; a full appraisal of how evidence-based healthcare is implemented in practice is discussed in Chapter 28).
- *Step 5: Evaluate the results.* Here it is crucially important to audit any changes in patient outcomes or service delivery as a result of changes made. This is to ensure that any perceived encouraging effects can be sustained and any harmful effects addressed and prevented.
- *Step 6: Disseminate the results.* Nurses are able to make substantial changes to patient care as a result of their EBP but sometimes they forget to share their knowledge with others. Part of the whole process is to disseminate knowledge to help others benefit from it.

The National Collaborating Centre for Methods and Tools has devised a useful resource and define a number of steps for EBP (specifically with public health in mind but arguably applicable to other areas of health), including

Define, Search, Appraise, Synthesise, Adapt, and Implement and Evaluate (https://www.nccmt.ca).

Chapter 21 provides details on how to use practical methods for disseminating evidence to others, from report writing to delivering a paper at a conference.

Conclusion

The ideal is that the combination of up-to-date best evidence from well-planned studies, health professional expertise and lived experience can facilitate optimum evidence-based care. EBP and EIDM are the hallmarks of professional care and the quest by successive governments to deliver the highest quality care at the optimum cost is likely to drive the profession towards seeking an improved evidence base to underpin and justify its practice. Glasper (2010) has indicated that the old adage 'that in God we trust, all others must bring data' applies just as much to the profession of nursing as it does to medicine. Measurement is a central principle of EBP and accurate measurement enhances decision making in all aspects of healthcare.

References

Bick, D. and Graham, I. (2010) *Evaluating the Impact of Implementing Evidence-Based Practice*. Wiley-Blackwell, Oxford.

Fineout-Overholt, E., Melnyk, B.M. and Schultz, A. (2005) Transforming health care from the inside out: advancing evidence-based practice in the 21st century. *Journal of Professional Nursing*, **21** (6), 335–344.

Glasper, E.A. (2010) Can high-impact nursing actions result in enhanced patient care? *British Journal of Nursing*, **19** (6), 1056–1057.

Harvie, D. (2002) *Limeys. The True Story of One Man's War Against Ignorance, the Establishment and the Deadly Scurvy*. Sutton Publishing, Stroud, UK.

Kaptchuk, T.J. and Kerr, R.E. (2004) Commentary: unbiased divination, unbiased evidence, and the patulin clinical trial. *International Journal of Epidemiology*, **33** (2), 247–251.

McDonald, L. (2001) Florence Nightingale and the early origins of evidence-based nursing. *Evidence Based Nursing Notebook*, **4**, 68–69.

Melnyk, B.M., Fineout-Overholt, E., Stillwell, S. and Williamson, K.M. (2009) Evidence-based practice: step by step: igniting a spirit of inquiry. *American Journal of Nursing*, **109** (11), 49–52.

Melnyk, B.M., Fineout-Overholt, E., Stillwell, S. and Williamson, K.M. (2010) Evidence-based practice: step by step: the seven steps of evidence-based practice. *American Journal of Nursing*, **110** (1), 51–53.

National Collaborating Centre for Methods and Tools. Evidence-informed public health. https://www.nccmt.ca/about/eiph (accessed 24 April 2020).

National Institute for Health Research. Clinical Research Strategy 2017–2020. Available at https://www.nihr.ac.uk/documents/nihr-clinical-research-nurse-strategy-2017-2020/11503 (accessed 24 April 2020).

Nursing and Midwifery Council (2018) *The Code: Professional Standards of Practice and Behaviour for Nurses, Midwives and Nursing Associates.* Nursing and Midwifery Council, London.

Parahoo, K. (2014) *Nursing Research, Principles, Process and Issues*, 3rd edn. Palgrave Macmillan, Basingstoke, UK.

Reid, S. (2008) Nothing new under the sun. *Evidence-Based Mental Health*, **11** (2), 33–34.

Sackett, D.L., Rosenberg, W.M.C. and Haynes, R.B. (1997) *Evidence Based Medicine. How to Teach EBM.* Churchill Livingstone, Edinburgh.

Stolberg, H.O., Norman, G. and Trop, I. (2004) Fundamentals of clinical research for radiologists. *Randomised controlled trials. American Journal of Roentgenology*, **183**, 1539–1544.

For further resources for this chapter visit the companion website at

www.wiley.com/go/glasper/nursingdissertation2e

Chapter 4 What is evidence-based practice and clinical effectiveness?

Andrée le May
University of Southampton, UK

Scenario

Regardless of the course they're doing, Sue, Alisha, Charlotte and Sam all need to think about how the decisions they make in practice are informed by evidence and that the care they give is effective.

This chapter is divided into three interlinked sections. In the first section, we consider the meaning of clinical effectiveness. In the second part the focus turns to evidence-based practice, a component of clinical effectiveness. In the third section we concentrate on how care may be made more effective.

Clinical effectiveness

What is clinical effectiveness?

Clinical effectiveness is about providing the best possible healthcare to people within the resources available. It is a term that has been used for over 20 years and is just as relevant today as it was in 1996 when the UK Department of Health defined it as:

> *The extent to which specific clinical interventions when deployed in the field for a particular patient or population do what they are intended to do, i.e.: maintain and improve health and secure the greatest possible health gain from the available resources.*

How to Write Your Nursing Dissertation, Second Edition.
Edited by Alan Glasper and Diane Carpenter.
© 2021 John Wiley & Sons Ltd. Published 2021 by John Wiley & Sons Ltd.
Companion website: www.wiley.com/go/glasper/nursingdissertation2e

That same year, the Royal College of Nursing (RCN) described clinical effectiveness as building on audit and quality improvement in order to provide a 'framework for linking research, implementation and evaluation in clinical practice' (Royal College of Nursing, 1996:3). This framework has more recently been portrayed, at a more personal level, by NHS Quality Improvement Scotland (2005) as:

the right person (you) doing:
- *the right thing (evidence-based practice)*
- *in the right way (skills and competence)*
- *at the right time (providing treatment/services when the patient needs them)*
- *in the right place (location of treatment/services)*
- *with the right result (clinical effectiveness/maximising health gain).*

Le May (2012:136–137) suggests that

in order to do this we need to:

- **have information available** *not only about the care that is being delivered – its effectiveness and efficiency – but also any new research evidence about the best care to provide and the best ways through which care could be delivered;*
- **openly scrutinise the delivery of care:** *practitioners, managers and support workers always need to be thinking about what they do and how they could do things better or more safely; this process needs to be logical and reviewed by others within the team providing health (and social) care – it is the opposite to practising traditionally or ritualistically, a criticism that is made of some nurses;*
- **include people who use health-care services in this process:** *service users are key drivers for clinical effectiveness, and it is important to try wherever possible to co-design services with them (Bates and Robert, 2006; Point of Care Foundation, https://www.pointofcare foundation.org.uk/). The Picker Institute published a set of eight principles related to patient-centred care that should be kept in mind when anyone is thinking about evidence-based practice and clinical effectiveness – it focuses on:*
  - *access to reliable advice*
  - *effective treatment*
  - *continuity of care*
  - *involvement of family and carers*
  - *clear information and support for self-care*

    ○ *involvement in decisions and respect for preferences*
    ○ *emotional support, empathy and respect*
    ○ *attention to physical and environmental needs.*

Activity 4.1

Access the Picker Institute website (https://www.picker.org/about-us/picker-principles-of-person-centred-care/) where you will find more information about each of these principles and a series of short video clips.

- ***identify where change is needed*** *and ensure that that change is based on evidence from research, examples of best practice from elsewhere or audit; change should be managed in a purposeful way to make its implementation as effective and efficient as possible;*
- ***ensure that all change is evaluated*** *to determine the extent of its success and altered if need be;*
- ***tell others about what has been done*** *either through publications or formal/informal presentations; failure to do this may be why information about the best care often fails to get across to everyone who needs to know and why care in some areas stagnates.*

This process needs to be done by everyone. Clinical effectiveness is not just the concern of those providing direct patient care, it needs to be the concern of their managers and their managers too; in other words... clinical effectiveness needs to be a concern of everyone in every organisation (or group of organisations) that provides health and social care.

Although thinking about clinical effectiveness and trying to make care more clinically effective are not new ideas, in reality clinical effectiveness can be hard to achieve. Difficulties are not only associated with the often-complex process of understanding care, evaluating its effectiveness and changing it when needed but also with resistance to change and feelings of discomfort when people believe that the care they have been given is effective when it is not.

In summary, clinical effectiveness comprises five key components.

1. Having *a way of thinking* that questions care delivery and makes everyone want to know how effective care has been for each person/group of people receiving it. This way of thinking will have started to develop during your initial nursing education, and of course is developing even now as you read this book! But once you have left your studies behind, it still needs to

continue to develop and be used to promote environments that encourage quality improvement.

2. Using *evidence usually from research or research-based guidelines* to support practice. This can be a challenge; there is so much evidence out there to select from, which interventions will be effective? A good place to start would be to check out the evidence collected on various databases (e.g. TRIP database http://www.tripdatabase.com/ or the Joanna Briggs Institute https://joannabriggs.org/) and any National Institute for Health and Care Excellence (NICE) (http://www.nice.org.uk/) or Scottish Intercollegiate Guidelines Network (SIGN) (http://www.sign.ac.uk/) guidelines related specifically to the care you are proposing to give. You need to appraise this evidence and decide if it is clinically relevant to your practice. (Chapter 6 gives more details on how to search for evidence-based literature.)

3. Having the *knowledge, skills and competence* to deliver that research-based care to patients appropriately (at the right time and in the right place); this includes trying to find out if the patient will stick to the prescribed care. From time to time the best research-based care does not work because we forget to tailor it to the patient's wider life and previous experiences. Sometimes, despite clear information and instructions, patients do not stick with the care we prescribe (e.g. leaving a particular dressing in place for a given length of time) because it does not suit them in some way. Understanding this – the 'burden' for them that care can create – is important in ensuring its success. If the effort of sticking to the care prescribed (e.g. living with side effects and restrictions on daily life) outweighs the benefits of that care, then the patient and their carers are likely to deviate from the care that is planned.

4. Having *an ability to evaluate practice* both at an individual level through evaluation of the success (or not) of daily care and at a group level through audit. This relies on setting clear outcome measures related to care: what do you, the patient and their carer(s) expect to achieve? These should be, wherever possible, shared objectives between the patient/carer and the multidisciplinary team. Only when you make the outcomes of care clear can care be measured in any meaningful way. Sometimes this measurement will rely on predetermined highly specific tools (e.g. the Edinburgh Postnatal Depression Scale, the SF-36 health measure or the MEWS/ NEWS2 early warning systems), sometimes it will depend on less structured observations of improvement (e.g. level of independence), and sometimes on much more qualitative data, in the form of patient stories for instance.

5. Having or developing *a commitment to disseminating* how effective care has been, and either formally or informally communicating this to others.

Activity 4.2

See the Mayo Clinic website (http://www.mayoclinic.org/patientstories/) and source a copy and read Gullick and Shimadry's (2008) paper in the *Nursing Times* (this can usually be accessed through your university learning resources centre's online resources, such as electronic journals and online databases).

In your study group discuss the implications and veracity of these patient stories.

Evidence-based practice

For well over 30 years, prominence has been given to the use of research evidence in healthcare in an attempt to further increase clinical effectiveness and the quality of care delivered to patients. Many definitions have been provided for evidence-based medicine/healthcare/practice but the one that best characterises the push for the use of research evidence in nursing comes from Cullum *et al.* (2008:2), who define evidence-based nursing as 'the application of valid, relevant research-based information in nurse decision making'.

Whilst noting the importance of applying valid and relevant research to practice, it is important to remember that rigorous and relevant research may not always be available to base practice on. If this is the case, practitioners need to consider what other sorts of evidence could be used to support effective and efficient care. Other sources of evidence might include:

- evidence based on structured evaluations of practice (audit or other analyses of safety records, complaints, etc.);
- evidence based on theory which is not grounded in research;
- evidence based on our experiences (professional and general);
- evidence gathered from our clients/patients and/or their carers;
- evidence passed on to us by role model experts;
- evidence based on policy directives.

All evidence, regardless of its source, needs to be critiqued. You will read more about critiquing research evidence in the subsequent chapters but don't forget to critique these other sorts of evidence too (see Table 4.1).

Sometimes none of these are relevant and we have to search more widely for knowledge to help us provide appropriate care. This might include searching for unpublished evidence in reports, research abstracts or conference proceedings using the internet or finding, as Sue has done in the scenario, information available in the media. Evidence emanating from the media needs particularly careful appraisal before implementation, with thorough follow-up of any primary sources referred to. If none are available you can check out any evidence base behind the article by using the website Behind the Headlines (http://www.nhs.uk/news/Pages/NewsIndex.aspx). This website gives you the 'facts without the fiction' and can be accessed by healthcare practitioners and patients. If you still need more information, contact the reporter.

Practising in an evidence-based practice way is usually described as a fairly simple linear process (Box 4.1). Of course, it is never as simple as it appears in theory and we discuss this in more depth in Chapter 5.

Attention needs to be paid to establishing the rigour of the evidence, research or otherwise. For research evidence this is primarily about reliability and validity. There are many guides and tools that can help you do this, for example the series of critical appraisal tools (CASP) available at the Centre for Evidence Based Medicine (CEBM; http://www.cebm.net/?o=1157) and advice is also provided in Sections 4 and 5 of this book. For other sorts of evidence le May and Gabbay (2011) have constructed a useful set of pointers (Table 4.1).

Once you've decided that the evidence is reliable and valid, it is important to establish its clinical relevance. This should be done by asking a set of questions (le May, 1999; le May and Gabbay, 2011) such as the following.

Is the evidence relevant clinically for the client?
1. What benefits will the implementation of this evidence have for patients/carers/staff?
2. What risks are associated with implementation/non-implementation?

Box 4.1   The process of evidence-based healthcare

1 Asking clear questions about practice, usually about an individual patient.
2 Looking for answers to those questions, firstly searching for research findings.
3 Judging (critically appraising) the evidence for its rigour, validity (truthfulness) and usefulness to practice.
4 Integrating these findings with clinical expertise, patient needs, and patient preferences.
5 If appropriate, applying these findings to the patient's care.
6 Evaluating the outcome of our decisions/practice.

Source: adapted from Sackett *et al.* (2004).

Table 4.1 Assessing the rigour of evidence: some initial elements for consideration.

Own experiences	Theoretical perspectives (non-research based)	Client's/patient's/carer's experiences	Role model's/expert's opinions	Policy directives
Relevance to the clinical issue	Link between theory and clinical issue	Relevance to the current situation	Depth and breadth of expertise	Type and strength of evidence used to support directive(s)
Frequency/uniqueness of experience	Strengths and weaknesses of argument being presented	Frequency/uniqueness of experience	Credibility	Relevance to current situation or clinical issue
Extent to which experiences have been shared by others	What sources of evidence are used?	Extent to which experiences have been shared by others	Reason for choice: what defines expertise?	Currency: date when last reviewed
Extent to which other sources of evidence support experiences	Credibility	Extent to which other sources of evidence support experiences	What sources of evidence are drawn upon to support knowledge?	Likelihood of transferability to practice setting
Extent of transferability of experiences to current situation	Appropriateness of theory to clinical issue	Richness of the description	Relevance of advice to current situation	Evidence of use elsewhere or evaluation of impact
	Appropriateness of recommendations for practice	Extent of transferability of experiences to current situation	Likelihood of transferability of evidence to practice setting	
	Likelihood of transferability to practice setting		Evidence of use elsewhere or evaluation of impact	
	Evidence of use elsewhere or evaluation of impact			

Source: adapted from le May and Gabbay (2011).

Can the evidence be used by the organisation within which care is being given?
1. Are there enough resources for implementation?
2. What are the opportunities for and constraints to implementing this evidence?

Once you have established that the evidence can be trusted and is clinically relevant to your client, then the implementation process can begin (see Section 6).

Making care more effective

Clinical effectiveness is embedded in our healthcare system, from the commissioning of services to the delivery of care. Earlier we said that clinical effectiveness had developed from audit and quality improvement; these links still remain, but it is also important to have the right evidence available as well as access to supportive organisational structures, for instance those supporting clinical governance. We will come back to the challenges faced by practitioners who are trying to get research into practice in Chapter 5.

There are many mechanisms already used for making care more effective – some are more directive and distant from the front line of care delivery than others. The more directive approaches include the following.

- Following guidance published by NICE, SIGN or a professional body such as the RCN or Royal College of Midwives (RCM). The extent to which care conforms to these guidelines may be measured through external audits in the form of inspections by the Care Quality Commission (http://www.cqc. org.uk/) or internal organisational audits.
- Through contractual incentives, for example Quality Outcomes Framework (QOF) of general practitioners' contracts. This awards points (and associated funding) to practices for achieving specific outcomes.
- Through regulation: the Nursing and Midwifery Council (NMC) sets standards/competencies against which practitioners deliver care.
- By monitoring care against explicit standards through organisational audits carried out by the Care Quality Commission with the purpose of promoting improvement in health and healthcare.

The less centrally directed ones tend to involve healthcare workers and service users in understanding the process of care, often described as the patient's journey through the healthcare system. These techniques have become increasingly sophisticated and systematised and have been given stranger and stranger names over the last 15 years! Some examples that you may be familiar with include the Deming Cycle, better known as the **P**lan, **D**o, **S**tudy, **A**ct (PDSA) cycle and Lean thinking. Originally developed from the car-making industry, they are now being successfully used in healthcare settings across the world to analyse and improve the process of care delivery and its outcome for patients (and staff). Despite using different methods (Box 4.2) they essentially aim to do one thing – help us determine if the care given to patients is as good as it possibly could be and, if not, provide us with ways to identify how care could be improved.

Chapter 4

Box 4.2   Summaries of the PDSA cycle and LEAN thinking

PDSA cycle

Popularised by the Institute for Healthcare Improvement (IHI; http://www.ihi. org/IHI/) in North America, the PDSA cycle has been used across the world in order to make improvements to healthcare. Essentially, it is about finding the answers to three key questions: What are we trying to accomplish? What change can we make that will result in an improvement? How will we know that a change is an improvement? The cycle is used to 'test a change by developing a plan to test the change (Plan), carrying out the test (Do), observing and learning from the consequences (Study), and determining what modifications should be made to the test (Act)' (http://www.ihi.org/IHI/ Topics/Improvement/ImprovementMethods/Tools/Plan-Do-Study-Act%20 (PDSA)%20Worksheet).

The PDSA cycle is most often associated with small-scale change at particular hotspots in an organisation or a particular care pathway. Although we often read about PDSA being used by healthcare workers, it can be effectively used by volunteers or lay carers. Maurice Wilson, a volunteer with the Healthy Communities Collaborative in Northampton, writes about what it was like to use the PDSA cycle to help change services within his local community. The collaborative used the PDSA cycle to place the onus for action on the community volunteers and by doing this enabled them

to work in equal partnership with health professions. The beauty of the project was that it was 'action-based', which meant success rested with community volunteers themselves: it was about people feeling included in any change and their contributions and opinions being valued (Wilson, 2005:127).

LEAN thinking

LEAN thinking is often described as a way of achieving larger-scale change across an organisation(s) and takes a somewhat different approach to the PDSA cycle. Refined by Toyota, this approach has been adapted for use in healthcare (Miller, 2005; Department of Health, 2008) but probably the best known use of LEAN thinking in nursing is the work undertaken on the 'Productive Ward' initiative supported by the Institute for Innovation and Improvement from 2007. LEAN thinking seeks essentially to do more with less (http://www.lean.org/), the emphasis being to strip out waste from the system so that care can be provided, to the highest possible standard, in the most cost-effective way. Various techniques are used within the LEAN thinking process (for a useful summary of these go to https://www.england.nhs.uk/improvement-hub/wp-content/uploads/sites/44/2017/11/Going-Lean-in-the-NHS.pdf).

Sometimes LEAN thinking is linked to Six Sigma, a very quantitative approach. Six Sigma has five phases: define, measure, analyse, improve and control (DMAIC). The first phase includes a cost–benefit analysis and only if this is acceptable should the project progress any further. In the measurement phase, baseline data are collected to help the project team understand and quantify what is happening at the outset. This information can then be used to design a solution which will improve care and produce measurable outcomes that will show success at subsequent monitoring (for more information go to http://www.isixsigma.com).

Making care more effective relies on everyone involved taking responsibility for its delivery, alteration and evaluation. This process needs to blend the systematic study of the process of care – either in one part of the organisation (e.g. the ward, the team or the unit) or across the organisation(s) (e.g. the hospital, the Trust, the health economy) – with evidence-based

Box 4.3 Tips for thinking about clinical effectiveness in your evidence-based practice healthcare dissertation/final project or evidence-informed decision-making assignment

- Emphasise how understanding your topic better could help improve clinical effectiveness.
- Make sure that if your question cannot be answered by finding research-based evidence on its own, you tell your readers what other sources of evidence you used to help you find out about your topic and how you appraised these pieces of evidence.

decision making. Whilst a range of quality improvement techniques is available to steer this process, undertaking it will also rely on some or all of the following:

- the provision of continuing educational opportunities following qualification;
- the use of skilled, inclusive leadership that engages everyone necessary;
- the harnessing of patients' and other lay representatives' views;
- the use of guidelines to guide and change practice;
- the use of local opinion leaders and champions;
- the allocation of protected time;
- the use of audit or other quality improvement techniques and feedback;
- the availability and use of profile-raising units, e.g. the Institute for Health Improvement in North America (http://www.ihi.org/IHI/), The Health Foundation in England (http://www.health.org.uk/);
- creating ways for people to meet in order to talk about practice and how to make it more effective.

References

Bates, P. and Robert, G. (2006) Experience-based design: from redesigning the system around the patient to co-designing services with the patient. *Quality and Safety in Health Care*, **15**, 307–310.
Behind the Headlines, http://www.nhs.uk/news/Pages/NewsIndex.aspx (accessed 26 February 2020).
Care Quality Commission, http://www.cqc.org.uk/ (accessed 26 February 2020).
CASP, http://www.cebm.net/?o=1157 (accessed 26 February 2020).
Cullum, N., Cilisha, D., Maynes, B. and Marks, S. (2008) *Evidence-Based Nursing: An Introduction*. Blackwell Publishing, Oxford.
Department of Health (1996) *Promoting Clinical Effectiveness: A Framework for Action in and Through the NHS*. The Stationery Office, London.
Department of Health (2008) *High Quality Care for All: NHS Next Stage Review Final Report*. The Stationery Office, London.
Gullick, J. and Shimadry, B. (2008) Using patient stories to improve quality of care. *Nursing Times*, **104** (10), 33–34.
Institute for Health Improvement, http://www.ihi.org/ (accessed 26 February 2020).
Joanna Briggs Institute, https://joannabriggs.org/ (accessed 26 February 2020).
le May, A. (1999) *Evidence Based Practice. Nursing Times Clinical Monograph No 1*. EMAP, London.
le May, A. (2012) Evaluating care. In: A. le May and S. Holmes, *Introduction to Nursing Research: Developing Research Awareness, chapter* 11. Routledge, London.

le May, A. and Gabbay, J. (2011) Evidence-based practice: more than research needed? In: G. Lewith, J. Cousins and H. Walach (eds) *Clinical Research in Complementary Therapies, chapter* 20. Churchill Livingstone Elsevier, Edinburgh.

Mayo Clinic, http://www.mayoclinic.org/patientstories/ (accessed 26 February 2020).

Miller, D. (2005) *Going Lean in Health Care.* Institute for Healthcare Improvement, Cambridge, MA.

National Institute for Health and Care Excellence, http://www.nice.org.uk/ (accessed 26 February 2020).

NHS Quality Improvement Scotland (2005), http://www.clinicalgovernance.scot.nhs.uk/section2/definition.asp (accessed 16 October 2010).

Picker Institute, https://www.picker.org/about-us/picker-principles-of-person-centred-care/ (accessed 26 February 2020).

Point of Care Foundation, https://www.pointofcarefoundation.org.uk/ (accessed 26 February 2020).

Royal College of Nursing (1996) *Clinical Effectiveness.* RCN, London.

Sackett, D., Strauss, S., Richardson, W. *et al.* (2004) *Evidence Based Medicine: How to Practice and Teach EBM.* Churchill Livingstone, London.

Scottish Intercollegiate Guidelines Network, http://www.sign.ac.uk/ (accessed 26 February 2020).

The Health Foundation, http://www.health.org.uk/ (accessed 26 February 2020).

TRIP database, http://www.tripdatabase.com/ (accessed 26 February 2020).

Wilson, M. (2005) Preventing falls in older people. In: M. Rawlins and P. Littlejohns (eds) *Delivering Quality in the NHS.* Radcliffe, Oxford.

For further resources for this chapter visit the companion website at
www.wiley.com/go/glasper/nursingdissertation2e

Chapter 5 **The challenges of delivering practice based on best evidence (in primary, secondary and tertiary settings)**

Andrée le May
University of Southampton, UK

> **Scenario**
>
> Sue, Alisha, Charlotte and Sam have all thought about what evidence-based practice means to them and what constitutes best evidence. Now they all need to think about making their everyday practice evidence based.

Chapter 4 of this book emphasised the importance of clinical effectiveness and evidence-based practice. This chapter considers the challenges of delivering practice based on the best available evidence. The chapter is divided into three sections: the first reminds readers that practice is underpinned by many sorts of evidence; the second details the barriers that may well stop practitioners, regardless of their clinical speciality, from using research evidence in their practice; and the final section identifies ways through which the use of research-based practice can be encouraged and suggests ways to overcome some of the known barriers to research implementation.

An evidence base for practice

Every nurse needs to make every effort to use, as Cullum *et al.* (2008:2) put it, 'valid, relevant research-based information in (their) decision making', since delivering research-based care is central to achieving clinical effectiveness. However, doing this is not as simple as it may at first appear. This may

How to Write Your Nursing Dissertation, Second Edition.
Edited by Alan Glasper and Diane Carpenter.
© 2021 John Wiley & Sons Ltd. Published 2021 by John Wiley & Sons Ltd.
Companion website: www.wiley.com/go/glasper/nursingdissertation2e

sometimes be because there simply is no research-based information available and other sorts of information have to be used, or the research evidence exists but cannot be found or if it can be found it cannot be used because it does not fit with patients' preferences or because the healthcare organisation does not have the necessary resources to implement it. Any or all of these factors may be further complicated by a process whereby research-based information is melded with other sorts of information, rendering its original state unidentifiable (Gabbay *et al.*, 2003; le May, 2009). This transformation makes it not only hard for practitioners to identity and articulate specific research findings that have informed their practice but also for others interested in the implementation of research to work out how much research is actually being used.

We can be sure, though, from research and from listening to nurses, that in the complex reality of practice nurses do not only use research-based information to guide their practice; they use many sorts of evidence in order to provide high-quality care (le May, 1999). More specifically, Rycroft-Malone *et al.* (2004) outlined four types of evidence that underpinned the delivery of care: research, clinical experience, patient experience and information from the local context. A year later Estabrooks *et al.* (2005) expanded this list by demonstrating, through two case studies, that nurses' practical knowledge was obtained from their social interactions with others, their experiences, documents and a priori knowledge. Additionally, Estabrooks *et al.* (2005:460) suggested that these findings challenged the 'disproportionate weight that proponents of the evidence-based movement ascribe to research knowledge'. A few years later, in a survey of 590 Australian general practice nurses Mills *et al.* (2009) found that experiential learning and interactions with clients, peers, medical practitioners and specialist nurses were of greater importance to their practice than knowledge found in research journals.

In opposition to this view Profetto-McGrath *et al.* (2007) found that whilst Canadian clinical nurse specialists accessed and used evidence from many sources, they indicated that research literature was a primary source of evidence and research was used in their decision making, with the choice of evidence often depending on the type of question they were answering. In addition to evidence gathered from 'front-line' nurses, healthcare team members and families, the clinical nurse specialists used the internet to search research databases and other online sources of evidence as well as using it to communicate with peers and ask questions about current practice. Gerrish *et al.*'s (2008) survey of nurses in two hospitals in England found that they, too, relied heavily on personal experience and communication with colleagues rather than formal sources of knowledge. However, they also found differences in levels of seniority, with the more senior nurses being more confident generally in accessing research and changing practice. This may well support Profetto-McGrath *et al.*'s (2007) positive findings about clinical nurse specialists, the two studies together suggesting that the more senior the practitioner the more able they are in seeking out research-based information and implementing change based on it. All these findings reflect the realities of practice experienced by many nurses today.

The findings from Gabbay and le May's (2004, 2011) ethnographic observations of GPs, practice nurses and medical students throw further light on the conundrum of research use in practice, showing that, and explaining how, practitioners bring together many types of knowledge in order to form a very broad evidence base for high-quality care; they called this amalgam 'clinical mindlines'. Clinical mindlines are:

> *internalised, collectively reinforced and often tacit guidelines that are informed by clinicians' training, by their own and each others' experience, by their interactions with their role sets, by their reading, by the way they have learnt to handle the(ir) conflicting demands, by their understanding of local circumstances and systems, and by a host of other sources . . . Clinicians build up mindlines as a bank of personalised, flexible syntheses of all the different types of theoretical and experiential knowledge that they need to be able to call upon instantaneously.*
> (Gabbay and le May, 2011:43–44).

Gabbay and le May (2004) also found that practitioners only briefly 'grazed' the research literature, paying minimal attention to this source of evidence as a way of informing their practice. This does not mean that practice was poor – on the contrary, care was excellent in the practices observed – neither does it mean that decisions were not based on research-based information; rather it may simply mean that research journals are not the main ways through which practitioners find out about research.

Barriers to the use of research evidence in practice

Over the last five years more emphasis has been placed by the UK government, the Higher Education Funding Council, the Department of Health and Social Care and research funders on the need to increase the impact of research 'at the bedside' in order to improve patient care and justify their considerable financial investment in research. Despite a concomitant effort to make research more readily available in guidelines and policy statements, many practitioners would agree, if asked, that nursing decisions are still not always informed by the best and most up-to-date research. But why is this so?

Chapter 5

Numerous researchers have tried to answer this question, hoping that by identifying barriers to research use they will be able to construct suitable interventions to promote better use of research. Let us take a look at what these barriers are.

Kajermo *et al.* (2010) brought together data from 63 research studies that have used the BARRIERS scale to assess barriers to nurses' research use over the last 20 years. This systematic review concludes that the main barriers are related to the setting within which implementation occurs and the presentation of research findings. The authors state that barriers were consistent over time and also location. More extensive qualitative data from a study of practitioners' and managers' cultures of research (le May *et al.*, 1998) suggested that whilst some barriers do revolve around the setting in which nurses work and the jargon used in the presentation of research findings (Box 5.1), there are other important factors, such as attitudes, beliefs and professional relationships, that need to be considered.

Box 5.1   Practitioners' perceived barriers to research-based practice

Attitudes
- Lack of cooperation
- Lack of motivation
- Fear
- Resistance to change/ritualised practice

Beliefs
- Research will not make a difference
- Research data are not appropriate
- Conviction that current practice is OK

Professional relationship
- Medical staff block implementation
- Medical staff consider nursing research substandard
- Nursing colleagues are uncooperative
- Senior staff are resistant to change
- Research should be undertaken by practitioners
- Research 'goes' with an individual
- Low grading of research staff

Organisational issues
- Time

- Pressure of workload
- Too much change

Educational issues
- Practitioners unaware of or unable to access research
- Lack of skills in critical appraisal
- Research reports are jargonistic

Source: adapted from le May *et al.* (1998).

Furthermore, Gerrish *et al.*'s (2008) survey showed distinct differences between junior and senior nurses. Whilst all 598 respondents said they were confident finding and using evidence in practice, the senior nurses not only felt more confident accessing various sources of evidence (e.g. published sources and using the internet) but were also confident initiating change. Conversely, junior nurses were less confident finding out about their organisation and were less confident implementing change. Lack of time and resources were also noted as major barriers by the more junior nurses but not their senior colleagues, who felt able to overcome these limitations. Barriers cited by clinical nurse specialists in Canada (Profetto-McGrath *et al.*, 2007) support previous research and included lack of time, lack of resources and lack of receptivity at both clinical and organisational levels.

There seems then to be some consistency emerging in relation to the barriers identified, with nurses' use of research-based information being affected by several tangible challenges associated with:

- their work setting (lack of receptivity at clinical and organisational levels);
- the way research findings are presented;
- lack of time;
- lack of/inappropriateness of resources.

These may also be influenced by their attitudes and beliefs about research and their own ability to implement change (le May, 2012).

In addition to the barriers detailed above, practitioners sometimes suggest that the wrong research is being done, as the results will not answer the questions that practitioners need answers to. Increasingly, efforts are being made to minimise this mismatch by strengthening interactions between practitioners and researchers in order to fine-tune research questions and designs to meet the needs of practice (le May, 2012).

Action research

One popular approach to doing this is to use action research which, as Sam explained to Sue over a coffee, is about 'engaging staff in research about their own practice enabling them to take ownership of the change'. Sam isn't the only one to think like this – Munten *et al.*'s (2010) review is testament to the increasing interest being paid to action research as a 'promising' mechanism for implementing evidence-based practice. Another approach is to develop Van de Ven and Johnson's (2006) idea of engaged scholarship, which closely links research to the needs of practice and policy through co-construction (Gabbay and le May, 2011; McCormack, 2011); this is rather like the idea of action research that excited Sam.

Encouraging the use of research evidence in practice

Knowing the barriers that nurses face in using research should make it easier to design interventions to help them. A quick search through the literature (le May, 2012) reveals that over the last 20 years many different approaches have been used to encourage nurses around the world to use research evidence in practice, with varying degrees of success. Given this huge literature a sensible way forward was to find a systematic review in order to provide conclusive evidence of which approaches were best.

Thompson *et al.*'s (2007) systematic review is the only one to focus on interventions aimed at increasing research use in nursing. They took a highly structured approach including only the most robust studies available. Although 8000 titles were screened only four studies met the criteria for inclusion, three randomised controlled trials and one controlled 'before and after' study. The principal intervention in all of the four studies was education but it was not just simply providing education that mattered, it was the way that the education was delivered that impacted on its success (or not). When education occurred in researcher-led educational meetings it was ineffective (two studies). However, when a local opinion leader led the educational meeting it was effective (one study) and when the education occurred in multidisciplinary committee meetings around a particular topic (oncology pain) it was also effective (one study). Unfortunately, the restrictive methodology of this systematic review only allows us to say that in some cases education works, in other cases it does not: what it does suggest is that education associated with an environment within which trusted colleagues are present (either as opinion leaders or multidisciplinary team co-workers) may make it more successful.

Education was also an important feature for Profetto-McGrath *et al.*'s (2007) sample of clinical nurse specialists in Canada along with peers and organisational support. Organisational support, interprofessional relation-ships and education also featured in le May *et al.*'s (1998) study of nurses and their managers in England; however, so did other interesting factors, namely reorganisations in the NHS and the creation of new structures/fora (Box 5.2).

In relation to these last two points, several reorganisations of the NHS have occurred since that study was completed, with the emergence of new structures that have offered many opportunities for the development of closer links between researchers and practitioners (le May, 2012). Probably the most ambitious of these is the Collaborations for Leadership in Applied Health Research and Care (CLAHRC) initiative developed in 2008, now known ad ARCs (Applied Research Collaborations), by the National Institute

---

Box 5.2 Opportunities to develop research-based practice

Organisational support
- Specific research and development strategy for Trust or for nursing
- Enhanced links with education providers
- Funding for courses and workshops; award schemes
- Specific appointments
- Identification and support of champions for nursing

New 'structures'
- Research fora
- Research awareness groups
- Proactive research/ethics committees
- Research centre
- Nursing development units

Interprofessional relationships
- Multiprofessional initiatives, e.g. guideline development
- Multidisciplinary research

Changing individuals
- Greater uptake of continuing education
- Recognition of importance of research by individuals
- Project 2000 and degree courses increasing individual skills and knowledge

Reorganised NHS
- Evidence-based purchasing

Source: adapted from le May *et al.* (1998).

for Health Research (NIHR) at the Department of Health in response to the Cooksey Report (Cooksey, 2006). CLAHRC's and ARC's primary functions are to conduct high-quality applied health research, implement findings from research in clinical practice, and increase the capacity of NHS organisations to engage with and apply research including continuing professional development (https://clahrcprojects.co.uk/about and https://www.nihr.ac.uk/explore-nihr/support/collaborating-in-applied-health-research.htm).

Alongside this, le May (2012) reminds us that there has been the almost parallel development of structures within the NHS and the higher education sector that gave rise to creation of formal Clinical Academic Career pathways (UKCRC, 2007; NIHR 2020). Another initiative spearheaded by the NIHR to promote closer links between research and practice encourages practitioners to stay in practice and develop their research skills by splitting their workload between delivering care and researching it. This initiative supports the already established nursing and midwifery consultant posts which have the remit, although not as explicitly detailed, to link closely the implementation of research with providing care.

Some researchers, practitioners and academics have put forward models or frameworks which, if followed, might improve the use of research-based information in practice. Probably the best known of these are the models developed and refined over the last 10 years by a team of researchers originally at the Royal College of Nursing in the UK – the Promoting Action on Research Implementation in Health Services (PARiHS) framework (Kitson *et al.*, 1998) – two Canadian teams working to produce the Ottawa Model of Research Use (OMRU) (Logan and Graham, 2010) and the Knowledge-to-Action (KTA) model (Graham and Tetroe, 2010), and the Australian Joanna Briggs Institute (Pearson, 2010). The main elements of these models are presented in Boxes 5.3–5.6, and further details of these and several other models and frameworks for implementing evidence-based practice are presented in a comprehensive textbook edited by Rycroft-Malone and Bucknall (2010).

Box 5.3 The main elements of the most recent Promoting Action on Research Implementation in Health Services (PARiHS) framework

1 This framework emphasises that the success of implementation depends on the relationship between key factors:

  (a) the nature of the evidence (whether it is research, clinical experience or patient experience)

  (b) the context within which it is implemented (this includes the culture of the organisation, leadership and the potential for evaluation)

(c) the ways through which this implementation is facilitated (this depends on the role of the facilitator and their attributes and skills).

2 The most successful implementation will occur 'when evidence is scientifically robust and matches professional consensus and patients' preferences . . . the context receptive to change with sympathetic cultures, strong leadership, and appropriate monitoring and feedback systems . . . and, when there is appropriate facilitation of change with input from skilled external and internal facilitators' (Rycroft-Malone, 2010:112–113).

3 This framework may be used to diagnose the receptiveness of each context to change and thereby tailor any facilitation to meet the needs of that specific context.

Box 5.4 The main elements of the Ottawa Model of Research Use (OMRU)

1 This model specifically focuses on getting valid research findings implemented.

2 There are six key structural elements:
   (a) the research-informed innovation
   (b) the potential adopters
   (c) the practice environment
   (d) implementation interventions for transferring the research findings into practice
   (e) the adoption of the innovation
   (f) the outcomes – health related and others.

3 In addition, there are three process elements (AME) that need to be considered:
   (a) assessment of barriers and supports (these are associated with structural elements a–c above)
   (b) monitoring how the research-informed innovation is implemented
   (c) evaluation of the impact of the innovation (monitoring and evaluation are linked closely to structural elements d–f above).

4 This model can be applied to evidence-based practice projects and also quality improvement projects.

In addition to these frameworks, Baker *et al.*'s (2010) systematic review of 26 studies of interventions that could successfully overcome barriers to change shows us how difficult it is to identify, with any degree of certainty, interventions that really do work. Whilst they indicated that tailored

Chapter 5

Box 5.5 The main elements of the Knowledge-to-Action (KTA) framework

This framework is conceptually robust, being derived from an analysis of 31 planned action/change theories in health and social sciences, education and management.

1 The framework emphasises the importance of social interaction and of tailoring evidence to meet contextual and cultural needs.

2 The framework comprises a number of phases:
   (a) identify problem/select knowledge
   (b) adapt knowledge to the local context
   (c) assess barriers to knowledge use
   (d) implement tailored intervention
   (e) monitor knowledge use
   (f) evaluate outcomes (both those associated with the process of change and the outcomes in relation to healthcare)
   (g) sustain knowledge use.

Box 5.6 The main elements of the Joanna Briggs Institute (JBI) framework for implementing evidence

This framework is particularly focused on the use of research evidence.

1 At its core there are four key components:
   (a) healthcare evidence generation
   (b) evidence synthesis
   (c) evidence/knowledge transfer
   (d) use of evidence.

2 Our primary concern is the use of evidence: this part of the framework focuses on practice change, embedding evidence through system/organisation-wide change and evaluating its impact.

3 The framework emphasises that the process of use of evidence is influenced by:
   (a) resources
   (b) education/expertise
   (c) patient preference
   (d) the availability of research
   (e) staffing levels, skill mix
   (f) policies.

interventions could change professional practice, they could not tell us which ones would be the most effective approaches to reducing barriers to change.

A good reference to read more about cross-cutting healthcare issues, and the advantages and challenges of implementing evidence in practice, is Greenhalgh (2017).

Conclusion

Whilst acknowledging that nurses and other healthcare professionals use many types of evidence to underpin effective practice, this chapter has emphasised the importance of research evidence. Implementing research-based information is not as easy as it first appears and the smooth flow of research into practice is often prevented by a series of individual and organisational barriers. However, there is an emerging body of knowledge which suggests that carefully targeted educational interventions, particularly those involving trusted colleagues and/or opinion leaders, may help to overcome some of these barriers. In addition, using participative research designs (e.g. action research) or engaged scholarship, which forges partnerships between researchers and practitioners, can also facilitate a closer match between the research needs of practitioners and the research generated for implementation. The whole process of research use may be structured by one of the many frameworks available. Using one of these frameworks may be helpful when you either come to change practice in your workplace or plan how you might undertake a change to practice, based on the answer to your question, in your dissertation.

References

Baker, R., Camosso-Stefinovic, J., Gillies, C. et al. (2010) Tailored interventions to overcome identified barriers to change: effects on professional practice and health care outcomes. *Cochrane Database of Systematic Reviews* (3), CD005470.

Cooksey, D. (2006) *A Review of UK Health Research Funding*. HMSO, Norwich.

Cullum, N., Cilisha, D., Maynes, B. and Marks, S. (eds) (2008) *Evidence-Based Nursing: An Introduction*. Blackwell Publishing, Oxford.

Estabrooks, C., Rutakumwa, W., O'Leary, K. et al. (2005) Sources of practice knowledge among nurses. *Qualitative Health Research*, **15** (4), 460–476.

Gabbay, J. and le May, A. (2004) Evidence-based guidelines or collectively constructed 'mind-lines'? An ethnographic study of knowledge management in primary care. *British Medical Journal*, **329**, 1013–1020.

Gabbay, J. and le May, A. (2011) *Practice Based Evidence for Healthcare: Clinical Mindlines*. Routledge, London.

Gabbay, J., le May, A., Jefferson, H. *et al.* (2003) A case study of knowledge management in multi-agency consumer-informed 'communities of practice': implications for evidence-based policy development in health and social services. *Health*, **7** (3), 283–310.

Gerrish, K., Ashworth, P., Lacey, A. and Bailey, J. (2008) Developing evidence-based practice: experiences of senior and junior clinical nurses. *Journal of Advanced Nursing*, **62** (1), 62–73.

Graham, I. and Tetroe, J. (2010) The Knowledge to Action framework. In: J. Rycroft-Malone and T. Bucknall (eds) *Models and Frameworks for Implementing Evidence-Based Practice: Linking Evidence to Action*. John Wiley & Sons, Chichester.

Greenhalgh, T. (2017) *How to Implement Evidence-Based Practice*. Wiley-Blackwell, Oxford.

Kajermo, K., Boström, A.-M., Thompson, D. *et al.* (2010) The BARRIERS scale: the barriers to research utilization scale. A systematic review. *Implementation Science*, **5**, 32.

Kitson, A.L., Harvey, G. and McCormack, B. (1998) Enabling the implementation of evidence based practice: a conceptual framework. *Quality in Health Care*, **7**, 149–158.

le May, A. (1999) *Evidence Based Practice. Nursing Times Clinical Monograph No. 1*. EMAP, London.

le May, A. (2009) Generating patient capital: the contribution of story telling in communities of practice designed to develop older people's services. *In: Communities of Practice in Health and Social Care*. Blackwell Publishing, Oxford.

le May, A. (2012) Evaluating care. In: A. le May and S. Holmes (eds) *Introduction to Nursing Research: Developing Research Awareness, chapter 10*. Routledge, London.

le May, A., Mulhall, A. and Alexander, C. (1998) Bridging the research–practice gap: exploring the research cultures of practitioners and managers. *Journal of Advanced Nursing*, **28** (2), 428–437.

Logan, J. and Graham, I. (2010) The Ottawa model of research use. In: J. Rycroft-Malone and T. Bucknall (eds) *Models and Frameworks for Implementing Evidence-Based Practice: Linking Evidence to Action*. John Wiley & Sons, Chichester.

McCormack, B. (2011) Engaged scholarship and research impact: integrating the doing and using of research in practice. *Journal of Research in Nursing*, **16** (2), 111–127.

Mills, J., Field, J. and Cant, R. (2009) The place of knowledge and evidence in the context of Australian general practice nursing. *Worldviews on Evidence-Based Nursing*, **6**, 219–228.

Munten, G., Van Den Bogaard, J., Cox, K., Garretsen, H. and Bongers, I. (2010) Implementation of evidence-based practice in nursing using action research: a review. *Worldviews on Evidence-Based Nursing*, **7**, 135–157.

National Institute for Health Research, https://www.nihr.ac.uk/documents/starting-a-clinical-academic-career-with-the-heenihr-ica-programme/22062 (accessed 28 February 2020).

Pearson, A. (2010) The Joanna Briggs Institute model of evidence-based health care as a framework for implementing evidence. In: J. Rycroft-Malone and T. Bucknall (eds) *Models and Frameworks for Implementing Evidence-Based Practice: Linking Evidence to Action*. John Wiley & Sons, Chichester.

Profetto-McGrath, J., Smith, K., Hugo, K., Taylor, M. and El-Hajj, H. (2007) Clinical nurse specialists' use of evidence in practice: a pilot study. *Worldviews on Evidence-Based Nursing*, **4**, 86–96.

Rycroft-Malone, J. (2010) Promoting Action on Research Implementation in Health Services (PARIHS). In: J. Rycroft-Malone and T. Bucknall (eds) *Models and Frameworks for Implementing Evidence-Based Practice: Linking Evidence to Action*. John Wiley & Sons, Chichester.

Rycroft-Malone, J. and Bucknall, T. (eds) (2010) *Models and Frameworks for Implementing Evidence-Based Practice: Linking Evidence to Action*. John Wiley & Sons, Chichester.

Rycroft-Malone, J., Seers, K., Titchen, A. *et al.* (2004) What counts as evidence in evidence-based practice? *Journal of Advanced Nursing*, **47** (1), 81–90.

Thompson, D., Estabrooks, C., Scott-Findlay, S. *et al.* (2007) Interventions aimed at increasing research use in nursing: a systematic review. *Implementation Science*, **2**, 15.

UKCRC (2007) *Developing the best research professionals. Qualified graduate nurses: recommendations for preparing and supporting clinical academic nurses of the future.* Report of the UKCRC Subcommittee for Nurses in Clinical Research (Workforce), United Kingdom Clinical Research Collaboration (UKCRC), London.

Van de Ven, A. and Johnson, P. (2006) Knowledge for theory and practice. *Academy of Management Review*, **31**, 802–821.

For further resources for this chapter visit the companion website at

🖰   **www.wiley.com/go/glasper/nursingdissertation2e**

Chapter 5

Section 2   **Sourcing and accessing evidence for your dissertation**

Sue asks Sam for advice. She has some ideal 'evidence' for her dissertation but it is from a Sunday supplement magazine; does this count as evidence, she asks? Sam tells her about the work of Professor Andrée le May. Charlotte, despite having learned the principles of searching electronic databases in her first year, has not been very adventurous with this since and has tended to rely on one database, Medline. She knows she needs to search more widely for her final assignment. For Alisha this is the first assignment of this nature and she is feeling a little overwhelmed so she and Charlotte decide to make an appointment with their subject librarian.

Chapter 6 **Sourcing the best evidence**

Diane Carpenter[1] and Alan Glasper[2]
[1]*University of Plymouth, UK*
[2]*University of Southampton, UK*

This chapter outlines the process of finding the best evidence through an effective literature search and by making the fullest use of all the help and support provided by your university library service.

Scenario

Sue and Sam are making a plan of action that includes gathering material for their dissertations and both Charlotte and Alisha need to find sources to complete their evidence-based practice assignments. Sue knows that there have been quite a lot of changes in the nursing section of the library since she last used it. Sam is used to accessing some information on the internet but is unsure of the best way of finding information on a particular topic that reaches the right academic standards to use in his dissertation. Charlotte was taught how to access electronic databases in her first year, but feels a bit rusty and for Alisha this is her first assignment of this nature. They decide the best way to equip themselves is by consulting their university nursing librarian and asking for some tips on what they should do if they are to collect good-quality articles for their dissertations.

Exploring and refining your question

As you can imagine, you cannot simply sit down in front of your computer, or stand in the library and start searching. You need to do a lot of important preparation first. So, before you start searching for papers and books you need to:

This chapter is based on an earlier chapter by Paul Boagy, Pat Maier and Alan Glasper

---

How to Write Your Nursing Dissertation, Second Edition.
Edited by Alan Glasper and Diane Carpenter.
© 2021 John Wiley & Sons Ltd. Published 2021 by John Wiley & Sons Ltd.
Companion website: www.wiley.com/go/glasper/nursingdissertation2e

- identify the topic of your research;
- identify the approach you are going to take;
- refine your question in order to target your research;
- identify key search words or phrases.

Identifying your topic

This is easy if you have a passion for something, but be careful that you clearly identify which part of a passionate topic you want to investigate. Always check that you will be able to find enough material on the topic. One area you can check is the National Institute for Health and Care Excellence (NICE) evidence search facility (https://www.evidence.nhs.uk). On this database you can search a topic, like 'heart attack', and find relevant articles related to this topic under diagnosis, economics, aetiology, prognosis, symptoms or therapy. Immediately you can see that saying that you want to do some research on 'heart attacks' means you need to refine it further.

Identify the approach you are going to take

Before you can start searching for your topic, you need to clearly understand what you are looking for within that topic. Some ways of looking at your topic are as follows.

- *The road map approach*: this traces the history of the topic and your work reviews its history. You will also have some critical reflection on what you review. You may want to investigate how patients with heart attacks have been treated over the last 20 years and what has influenced the changes in approach and the prognosis.
- *Here we go again*: this relates to people who are carrying out a research dissertation that includes gathering data, which many of you will not be doing. It involves the researcher using current knowledge and/or existing methodology and attempts to replicate, verify or refute previous results. They then discuss their results in light of previous work.
- *Can I prove it?* This is an experimental approach, again in research data-gathering dissertations, where the researcher sets up a hypothesis and attempt to disprove it. This approach may be linked to the 'Here we go again' approach.
- *The Swiss cheese approach*: you present current knowledge where the purpose is to show where there are gaps or holes in the field that require further attention or consideration.
- *Eyeball switch*: you look at existing research in the light of a new approach/theory. How can you re-interpret previous research with this new lens? You may want to look at therapies, diagnosis or symptoms that have been used in the past in the light of new knowledge, or apply a technique used

in one clinical setting to another where it has not currently been considered.

Take a closer look at these approaches and identify the approach that resembles yours the most. If it is not listed, then write your own approach.

Refine your research question

Once you have decided on the precise nature of your topic and the kind of approach you want to take, you can then ensure that your question is fully refined to enable targeted searching. Here are three points to consider to help with this process.

My aspect will be. . .

What aspect will you look at, for example diagnosis, economics, aetiology, prognosis, symptoms or therapy? Is there anything else not on this list? Sue, Sam, Charlotte and Alisha are beginning to refine their searches.

The scope of the patients will be. . .

If you are dealing with patients, can you further refine this and determine the scope of the patients you will deal with, for example gender, age, part of the country, those having undergone a particular intervention at a particular time? Is there anything else not on this list? Chapter 9 provides more detail on how to pose evidence-based practice questions.

I will be looking at. . .

If you are not dealing with patients, what are you dealing with, for example, hospital practice of a topic in a particular area, government policy, interprofessional working practices, and nursing attitudes? Do you want to limit the scope by identifying a particular clinical area, group of nurses? What else can you add to this list that applies to you?

Identify search words

Now you have refined your topic and its scope, you need to identify the search words that you will want to use in order to find appropriate research. Try to be as methodical as you can with this and remember that when you do come to search, you will need to take into account the variations in certain words, for example:

- use a word related to the one you have written down (a thesaurus may help you to find synonyms);
- consider variations in the word, for example noun, adjective, singular or plural (see 'truncation' and 'wildcard' later);

- try using both American and UK spelling;
- limit your phrase length in order to keep on target (only include key words in your phrase – it need not be grammatically correct).

Being aware of this is very important as you could miss some key references if you are not careful. You need to develop a method for identifying your key words; two ways of going about this are mentioned here. You may also develop your own way.

Using a mind map to identify your key words

One way is to produce a mind map either using mapping software (e.g. *Mind Manager* or *Inspiration*) or a large sheet of paper. Write the question in the centre of the paper, and then fill the rest of the sheet with as many other words, phrases, acronyms and so on as you can think of which relate to some aspect of the question. These words and phrases can then be grouped by using different coloured pens. Select one word or phrase on the sheet and mark it with one colour. Using the same colour pen, mark any other words or phrases that are related to this aspect of the question. Then select a second colour, choose an unmarked word or phrase on the sheet and repeat the process. If there are any remaining unmarked words and phrases, choose another colour and continue as before.

Using a linear figure to identify your key words

You can treat your question as a linear rectangle, divided into perhaps three or four sections, each section representing one aspect of the question. Taking each section in turn, list below it as many words or phrases as you can think of which relate to that aspect of the question.

Developing a methodical process will ensure that you systematically derive lists of key words and phrases that you can then use in your literature search. It will also give you something to return to if you need to revise your search strategy later on. The next step is to select the appropriate bibliographic databases for searching.

Searching for research articles

As part of a comprehensive search for evidence, you will need to undertake a thorough literature review. This involves identifying and evaluating the research journal articles which have been published on your topic. For this purpose you will need to have access to a range of bibliographic databases, such as CINAHL, British Nursing Index (BNI) or SCOPUS. Random browsing of the journals you happen to be aware of, or have been told about by colleagues, will help but will not be a sufficiently robust way of literature searching.

What are bibliographic databases?

Bibliographical databases are computer-based resources that provide references to the published journal literature and enable you to undertake comprehensive and systematic literature searches. Access to, and use of, these bibliographical databases assumes that you have the appropriate level of IT skills and the confidence to undertake the searching process on your own, making use of help and support where necessary.

Why we have bibliographic databases

Within their individual scope they offer a means of systematically identifying the journal and other types of literature that have been published in particular subject areas. Information on some of the most important databases covering the healthcare fields follows later.

> **Scenario**
>
> Sue and Sam have attended a lecture given by one of the librarians on how to search the literature. The librarian had made them laugh by describing libraries as being like the Albert Hall full from top to bottom with journal papers. Students cannot simply dive in and look for the only four papers ever published on the subject of larvae therapy for the treatment of foot wounds, as the chance of success would be statistically very small. What is needed to succeed, the students were informed, was to be systematic and use the university databases wisely.

Chapter 6

The function of bibliographic databases

Bibliographic databases provide references to articles published in journals and, in some cases, they also cover other types of literature, such as theses and dissertations, books and book chapters, government reports and policy documents. Updated on a regular basis, the databases are searchable in different ways and provide sophisticated techniques for developing and revising your searches. Some database providers offer the facility for you to store your searches on the system, enabling you to revisit and update your literature

> **Tip**
>
> if you do not know what current awareness services look like search for 'Current Contents/OVID' or simply search more generically for 'Current Awareness Services'. You may want to add 'Nursing' or 'Medical' to target your search.

searching as your work progresses. In some cases, current awareness services are also available for you to make use of. These services will provide automatic email alerts for you when new references that relate to your stored searches are added to the database.

How do the databases work?

The databases work by providing searching facilities to produce a list of references that can then be followed up. It is possible to search the databases in different ways – by subject keyword or phrase, author or title for example, or combinations of these. It is also possible to refine and restrict your search in a number of ways: by date of publication, type of publication, language or place of publication, for example, depending on the facilities offered by the particular database you are using.

A search will generate a list of articles that can then be stored, downloaded or printed off from the database. In some cases a list of the cited references may be available as part of the article record. This can be a useful way of finding further references on the topic in the early stages of your searching, as well as for triangulating your search methodology (i.e. cross-referencing from several search methods). The cited references are those books, articles and other resources which the authors themselves referred to while writing their article, and are usually provided as a list at the end of the article, with links from the text of the article concerned.

In the case of some bibliographic databases, direct links from the record to the full text of the article are sometimes available; if not, then your library and information service will provide access to a range of electronic and printed journals, or to document supply facilities in cases where the journal article you need is not held locally.

Getting access to the databases

Access will be provided by your library and information service, with links via their website; for NHS staff, they are currently provided by the electronic (NHS) Health Information Resources federated search facility. A federated search facility is a search engine that simultaneously searches multiple databases or web resources for you. This may sometimes be referred to as a web portal in your institution. If you are currently studying with a university, you can normally expect the databases to be available for you to use both on and off campus, via the library service's web pages.

Databases available to you

Within the healthcare field, there a number of large and powerful bibliographic databases that are widely used by researchers. Most of them include abstracts of the articles they reference.

- *Allied and Complementary Medicine Database* (AMED) is produced by the Health Care Information Service of the British Library. It is an important database for complementary medicine and palliative care. It is updated monthly.
- *Applied Social Sciences Index and Abstracts* (ASSIA) is an indexing and abstracting tool covering health, social services, psychology and sociology, among other subjects. It is updated monthly.
- *British Nursing Index* (BNI) indexes the most popular English-language nursing and related journals. It is updated monthly.
- *Cumulative Index to Nursing and Allied Health Literature* (CINAHL) is a comprehensive index to literature published worldwide. Over 2500 journals are currently indexed and other types of material, such as American doctoral dissertations, are also included. It includes some full text links and is updated weekly.
- *EMBASE* is a major biomedical and pharmaceutical database, indexing over 3500 international journals. It is updated weekly.
- The *Health Management Information Consortium* (HMIC) database includes references derived from two different sources: the Department of Health's Library and Information Services and the King's Fund Centre Information and Library Service. It is particularly useful for searching for references on health services policy and management, and indexes books, reports and journal articles; both parts of the database provide a useful means of identifying grey literature. It is updated bimonthly.
- *MEDLINE* is produced by the National Library of Medicine in the USA and is the most important biomedical database for literature searching. It indexes over 3900 journals published worldwide and is updated daily.
- *PsycInfo* is the main database for searching the literature of psychology, psychiatry and related fields. It includes references from as far back as 1806 up to the present, covering journal articles, books, chapters and dissertations. It is updated weekly.

Getting help in using the databases

Most of the databases have built-in help screens available and, in some cases, links to guide leaflets that can be printed off. You can also expect your library and information service to provide online or printed guide leaflets and help sheets and, in most cases, one-to-one help and group tutorials. If you have never used them before, these databases can sometimes appear daunting and even the experienced searcher will need to keep up with changes to them. It is always worth seeking out some help, as discussed later.

Chapter 6

Why it is not best practice to rely on Google

Google is easy and convenient to use but will not provide such a comprehensive and systematic survey of the literature as you will be able to achieve by using one or more of the databases outlined above. It is worth emphasising that best evidence is usually found in journal articles that have been peer reviewed, namely screened before publication by experts in the field. The main databases access peer-reviewed journals but Google does not discriminate in relation to the quality of evidence in this way; rather, it depends on availability rather than quality. It is, however, important to remember that the search engine Google Scholar is a very useful first stop for investigating the parameters of just what is available. Google Scholar is a citation index and may therefore not host the most up-to-date journal papers.

Devising your search strategy

Having identified the key terms and concepts that cover your research topic, and learned something of the bibliographic databases available for searching, you can then begin to devise your search strategy.

Subject searching: keyword or free text searching

A keyword or free text search means that you will be looking for every occurrence of a particular word or phrase, wherever it appears – normally in the title or abstract of the reference – within the record. This type of search is very wide and normally retrieves the largest possible number of records, but some of the references may appear less relevant to your subject. If you use this type of search, you will need to have considered all the possible synonyms for the same concept, for example 'youth', 'teenager', 'adolescent' and 'young adult', and then search the databases using each of the terms.

Using a subject thesaurus

The most important databases, such as CINAHL, MEDLINE and BNI for example, include a subject thesaurus. If you perform a search on the database using this facility, it will convert a word or phrase into the suggested main indexing term. Using this, you can gather together all the references included on the database which are indexed using the same term. This can be more effective than keyword searching if there are a number of different synonyms for your particular term. Using the example above, the CINAHL subject heading for all of these is 'Adolescence'; it is also possible to 'focus' on this subject heading, so that you retrieve a list of articles where this term is regarded as a major aspect of the articles concerned.

A search using truncation

All the databases also offer various other searching techniques, such as truncation and the use of wildcards. Truncation means that you can perform a keyword/free text search using a term such as *assess** (with a '*' character after the word), which looks for *assess, assessed, assessing, assessment* and so on, without having to search for all the different words separately.

Similarly, if you want to search for articles that contain *child, children, child's, children's, childhood*, then searching *child** will retrieve them all. However, it will also retrieve *childbirth* which is something you may not want in your particular context.

A search using wildcard

A wildcard search normally uses the '?' character, where there may be another letter present, for example *p?ediatric* which will search for both *paediatric* and *pediatric*.

A search using Boolean logic

This keyword/free text searching technique uses one of the Boolean operators AND, OR and NOT, named after the nineteenth century mathematician who devised the system of logical operations. Using the example above, you would specify *child** NOT *childbirth*.

Boolean terms

AND	finds articles that contain all of the search terms combined with AND
OR	finds articles that contain each of the search words, but not necessarily in combination with each other
NOT	excludes a word from the search, for example *child** NOT *childcare*.

A search using phrases

Most databases provide the facility to search for a word or phrase within the title of articles, which will give a shorter but much more focused list of references. Alternatively, you may have the name of a specific author and wish to search for all the papers written by that person. This is known as field searching, the fields being each different section of the database record.

Imposing restrictions on your search

You will also need to consider any possible limits and exclusions that you wish to incorporate in your search (for example, language, date of publication, type of material, specific methodologies).

Chapter 6

- *Language*: some of the literature searching databases include references to articles published globally, in many languages, and it can be very difficult to obtain translations if you are not proficient in the language concerned. You may wish to restrict your search to English-language articles only; this facility is usually provided.
- *Date*: you will also need to think about restricting your search by the date of publication if you wish to retrieve references published more recently or within a particular date range. The databases sometimes include references to articles published over a very long period and will not automatically do this for you, although most of them will usually display your references in reverse date order, showing the most recent publications first in the list. How far back in the literature you need to search will depend to some extent on the nature of the topic you are working with and on the available published literature. Otherwise there may have been a key research paper, policy document or report which changed the subsequent nature of the research on the topic and you may only want to find articles which have been published later than that.
- *Type of material*: if you are only searching for journal articles, you need to bear in mind that some of the databases also include references to other types of material. For example, PsycInfo includes references to books and book chapters, as well as to journal articles, and CINAHL includes references to American college and university dissertations. HMIC includes references to grey literature as well as journal articles. Grey literature is the collective term used to describe publications which originate in ways outside mainstream publication, such as academic theses, unpublished research reports, information produced for patients, and so on. Depending on the nature of your topic you may wish to include a search for this type of material. CINAHL enables you to limit your search to research articles or to evidence-based practice, for example. You need to remember, however, that the more of these specific limits you apply to a search, the fewer references you will retrieve.
- *Specific methodologies*: some of the databases enable you to include restrictions as to the type of methodology used in the research, such as provided by the Clinical Queries limit on MEDLINE.

The databases will display your search history. This will list each of the terms you have searched, indicating the number of references found in each case, and enabling you to combine different terms in the history if you wish.

If your search does not find anything or finds material not relevant
If you are unhappy with the list of references provided by your database search, you will need to revise your search. If you have not found any refer-

ences at all, check your spelling and typing. The databases will only search for what you have asked for! If the references seem too specific, revisit your original mind map or diagram and look for a more general term you can use instead. Alternatively, if the search results are too general, consider a more specific term and go back to the database.

Accessing journal literature

After you have done some searching, you will want to access the article itself. So how do you do that?

When you have undertaken a search of the appropriate databases for your subject, and retrieved a list of references, you need to decide which of the references you wish to follow up. Normally, where an abstract is provided as part of the record, this is sufficient to enable you to make this decision. Sometimes, however, if there is no abstract or the title of the article is unclear, you may need to read the article itself to know whether or not it is of relevance.

To trace a particular article, look at the reference's source details. This will indicate the journal in which the article was published, as well as giving you full bibliographic details (volume and/or issue number, date and pages), enabling you to trace the article.

Knowing which journals you can access

Your library and information service will provide access to journals, in a number of ways, and will enable you to check which ones are available. Access to the electronic full-text version of the journal from the library's web catalogue, or via a journal management system (such as TDNet), linked from the library's web pages, are the two most usual means of access provided by libraries.

Using the journals themselves in electronic full text on a computer, rather than in printed format, is now the accepted means of access, except for some older material and a small number of specialist titles. This changeover from print to electronic format has taken place very quickly over the last few years and is beneficial for the user in a number of ways. Among the greatest benefits are the ease of use and convenience of access, with many people now having access to the internet at home as well as at work. This reduces the amount of time needed to visit the library taking writing materials.

In most cases, it is straightforward to print off or download a copy of the article you need. However, you must always bear in mind the limits imposed by copyright legislation, which restricts printing or photocopying of one article from an individual issue of a journal.

Because of complicated licensing requirements, university libraries can only allow access to electronic journals for their own current students and staff. University libraries, in particular, have been able to provide access to very many more electronic full-text journals than were previously available for their users in printed format, because of the way that subscriptions and access to electronic resources has been coordinated at a national level.

e-Journals

Journals now provide their articles in electronic form and once you have searched and selected an article, you will be able to download that article onto your PC providing your institution subscribes to that journal. Increasingly, you will find that most of your articles will be available in this format.

Some literature searching databases include full-text links to articles from the database records. It is often better, however, to keep the two stages of the literature searching process separate, as things can sometimes get very confusing, especially if you are an inexperienced searcher and working with more than one database and search. Search for the literature first, then follow up by tracing the articles.

Printed journals

Those libraries that still retain printed journals will record their holdings in their web catalogue, or in the case of a small library service may perhaps produce a list of them. Of course, access to printed journals will usually necessitate a visit to the library itself, unless it can offer a service whereby photocopies of articles can be sent to you.

Inter-library requests

Quite often your literature searching will identify articles that have been published in journals that are not held by your library service or available to you on the computer. It is usually possible to obtain copies of these articles by using your library's inter-library request service. This is normally regarded as a special service, as significant costs may be involved, and you may find that there is a charge for using the inter-library service, or that your use of it is restricted.

The Cochrane Library

The Cochrane Library deserves its own section. It describes itself as the best single source of reliable evidence about the effects of healthcare.

Why is it so important?

As part of a search for the best evidence, it must be regarded as the most important resource for information about the effectiveness of healthcare treatments and interventions. A web-based resource, it is currently available free of charge and without the need for user registration. It is available through the Health Information Resources, and other types of library services provide links to it from their websites in support of their own users.

The Cochrane Library comprises a number of separate databases that may be searched together or individually.

- Cochrane Database of Systematic Reviews (Cochrane Reviews)
- Database of Abstracts of Reviews of Effects (Other Reviews)
- Cochrane Central Register of Controlled Trials (Clinical Trials)
- Cochrane Methodology Register (Methods Studies)
- Health Technology Assessment Database (Technology Assessments)
- NHS Economic Evaluation Database (Economic Evaluations)

The Cochrane Library also includes information about the Cochrane Collaboration, which is the international organisation involved with the work of the specialist Cochrane Review Groups, Methods Groups, Fields and Centres.

Chapter 6

What information does the Cochrane Library contain?
Each of the component databases of the Cochrane Library contains a different type of information, as follows.

Cochrane Database of Systematic Reviews (Cochrane Reviews)
Cochrane systematic reviews are the 'gold standard': the highest quality of reviews of research evidence. The database currently includes over 3500 completed reviews and more than 1800 protocols, which are reviews in progress. They deal with many different research questions. In each case, within the criteria set by the Cochrane reviewers, all the published research on the topic is assessed and evaluated using the most rigorous procedures. The aim is to determine whether or not there is conclusive evidence about the effectiveness or otherwise of the particular healthcare treatment or intervention under consideration. The completed reviews may subsequently be updated, or have comments added to them, or, in some cases, they may be withdrawn as the review becomes out of date. Any such amendments are clearly indicated in the review. For this reason, it is necessary to make a note of the particular edition of the Cochrane Library you searched. It is currently updated four times a year, and the latest edition is indicated on the main screen, with some of the new content listed. The list of reviews can be browsed in several different ways.

Database of Abstracts of Reviews of Effects (Other Reviews)
This database is produced by the Centre for Reviews and Dissemination at the University of York. It includes structured abstracts of quality-assessed reviews of research evidence from published journal literature; newly added abstracts are indicated. There are currently more than 5000 abstracts in this database.

Cochrane Central Register of Controlled Trials (Clinical Trials)
Next in the hierarchy of evidence provided by the Cochrane Library, this database includes references to randomised controlled trials which have been published in the research journal literature. The records are largely derived from the EMBASE and MEDLINE bibliographical databases. The individual references include abstracts but no links to the full text of the journal articles concerned. There is also material in the database which is provided by the Cochrane Review Groups themselves. The database contains approximately 500 000 records in total.

Cochrane Methodology Register (Methods Studies)
This specialist section of the Cochrane Library deals with the methodology of controlled trials and systematic reviews, and is produced on behalf of the Cochrane Methodology Review Group by the UK Cochrane Centre, which is currently part of the NHS R&D Programme, based in Oxford. It includes references to books, journal articles and conference proceedings.

Health Technology Assessment Database (Technology Assessments)
This database is produced by the Centre for Reviews and Dissemination. It brings together details of completed and continuing health technology assessments from around the world. It differs from the other sections of the Cochrane Library in that the abstracts it contains are descriptive rather than analytical.

NHS Economic Evaluation Database (Economic Evaluations)
The cost-effectiveness of health interventions and treatments is the focus of this part of the Cochrane Library. It is another product of the Centre for Reviews and Dissemination, and contains over 5000 references to quality-assessed economic evaluations.

Searching the Cochrane Library
The content of the Cochrane Library may be searched in a number of different ways. The individual databases can be searched separately or together. On the main page of the Cochrane Library there is a box for a basic search term, which will search for the term in titles, abstracts and keywords across the content of all the individual databases. This works well for a very specific

concept, or a named drug for example, but is ineffective for very general words such as 'pain'. Advanced searching allows more detailed searching within record titles, and on-screen help is available. MeSH searching is a third option and involves the use of a thesaurus of subject headings. This facility is also available on the MEDLINE database. More information about this technique is available on screens within the Cochrane Library.

Browsing the Cochrane Library

As an alternative to the searching techniques described above, it is also possible to browse some of the individual databases within the Cochrane Library.

The Database of Systematic Reviews can be browsed in several ways:

- topic
- new reviews and protocols
- updated reviews
- an A–Z list
- Cochrane Review Group.

The Cochrane Methodology Register (Methods Studies), the Health Technology Assessment Database (Technology Assessments) and the NHS Economic Evaluation Database (Economic Evaluations) may all be browsed alphabetically, with newly added entries indicated through the list. The Database of Abstracts of Reviews of Effects (Other Reviews) and the Cochrane Central Register of Controlled Trials (Clinical Trials) are both deemed too large to facilitate browsing, and advanced searching is offered as an alternative.

Getting help using the Cochrane Library

The Cochrane Library provides a comprehensive assortment of support information targeted at different user groups. There are links to this material from the main page, and it may be downloaded. There is information here for the new user as well as for the expert researcher. It is also worth asking your library service if they have produced a guide leaflet. If they have, then it is likely to be written in a way they know will assist their clients.

Chapter 6

Scenario

Like Charlotte, Alisha does not have to complete a dissertation, but she has been set an essay to demonstrate that she can search for and find useful research-based literature. She needs to select a topic, formulate a question, search three databases, and demonstrate using inclusion and exclusion criteria how she will identify five articles that should be worth critical appraisal. At this stage, however, she has no idea at all what topic to select so has asked Anna (the subject librarian for healthcare) to help.

ALISHA   I'm sorry Anna I keep going round in circles and can't decide which topic to select.

ANNA   Don't worry, this is more common than you think. One good way to get inspiration is to browse the Cochrane Library. If you identify a Cochrane review you will be able to see how recently a topic has been studied. If you find a very recent systematic review, then you might select it for critical appraisal; however, you might also have difficulty finding other studies that are not already included in the review. If you find a Cochrane review that is a few years old, you should be more likely to find subsequent research studies that you could also select to appraise. I'll leave you for a few minutes to browse. . .

ANNA   How did you get on?

ALISHA   It's fascinating. I looked under complementary and alternative therapies, because I have an interest in that. I found a review that had been undertaken in 2017 about vitamin E for use in Alzheimer's disease and mild cognitive impairment (Farina *et al.*, 2017). I wondered whether it might be too recent so I searched on Medline and there do not seem to be any similar studies that are more recent so I guess I'll just have to go back to the drawing board, but I can see how to go about it now, thank you.

Activity 6.1

Try this for yourself. Browse the Cochrane Library for a topic heading, click on it and look at the systematic reviews that have been completed in that field. Then check against another database to see whether you can find additional articles that have not been included in the Cochrane review.

Websites and other resources

The internet has now become the accepted way for many people beginning a search for information. Access to the internet at home, as well as at work, or using the local public library, or university or college networks, is now a reality, and it is possible to have access to knowledge on a global scale.

The amount of accessible information can be bewildering, if not overwhelming, and you need to be able to navigate your way through it all. In particular, you need to be able to distinguish the good from the bad (or downright misleading, or even dangerous). Great care must be taken to ensure that you only use information from quality assured, authoritative and up-to-date sites.

Evaluation of websites

One of the most important websites currently available to you is the Health Information Resources, which is a comprehensive electronic library and information service provided for the National Health Service. This encompasses a very wide range of information resources, guidance and specialist advice tailored for the health practitioner. It includes direct links to other evidence-based resources, such as the Cochrane Library, as well as to sources of clinical guidance and of images, and also to some of the bibliographic databases discussed earlier. As the working library for the National Health Service, it also provides password-controlled access to a range of electronic journals, electronic books and databases. It is searchable in a number of different ways and detailed online assistance is provided.

Important features of the Health Information Resources are the specialist libraries, which gather together the resources within a number of major clinical areas, such as cancer, diabetes and stroke for example, as well as some generic areas, such as women's health and child health. The search facility within each of the specialist libraries encompasses not only evidence and guidance but also some types of grey literature, such as reports and policy documents, learning materials, information on organisations, conferences and courses, as well as patient-related information.

The specialist libraries also offer an effective way of keeping up to date with new material as it becomes available, with current awareness and alerting services.

Support from your library service

If you are currently working in the National Health Service, or are studying at a university or college, you will have access to a library and information service, which perhaps you may not have used very much in the past. The library has a crucial part to play in supporting your dissertation work by providing the resources and facilities you will need.

There are a number of different types of library:

- those provided by National Health Service Trusts;
- academic libraries, provided by universities and colleges;
- public libraries;
- information services in other types of organisation, which may be provided by an information specialist working as part of a multiprofessional team;
- libraries provided by professional organisations such as the Royal College of Nursing (RCN);
- charitable trusts and foundations, such as the King's Fund Centre.

The way the library and information service is delivered will differ in some respects in each case, for example regarding the amount of individual assistance it is possible to provide for users and the availability of library resources.

You may be able to access a number of different library services, across different sectors, depending on your circumstances at the time, as long as you conform to the membership requirements of the particular library. On the other hand, you may find it more convenient and beneficial to use one particular library, and to develop a close relationship with the service and with the staff who can assist you.

If you currently work in the NHS, you can find details of your local NHS library by searching the Health Library and Information Services Directory website (http://www.hlisd.org/, last accessed 14 January 2020). This currently provides details of more than 1300 library and information services, and is searchable by library or staff name, or geographically by place or postcode.

The assistance you will receive from your library/information service will include:

- making available a selection of textbooks, to enable you to read around your research topic for background information;
- providing printed journals, reports, official documents, dvds/videos and other types of material, as well as access to electronic information resources such as databases and journals via the internet;
- helping and advising with all stages of the literature searching process and document delivery;
- training in information skills, on a one-to-one basis and in groups;
- updating you on changes to information resources and services;
- providing face-to-face, email and web-based enquiry services;
- providing an inter-library service for books and journal articles not held locally;
- accessing detailed information via the library service's web pages;
- troubleshooting, when you are really stuck!

Each type of library strives to provide an efficient and effective service within the scope of its available resources. Now is the time to get to know your library and make the most of what it has to offer.

This is an important point. Sometimes we can become very wedded to our topic of interest, but for one reason or another may not find a sufficient number of studies to critique. If this occurs we need to check our search terms and synonyms first and consider whether we have selected the correct databases.

Scenario

Charlotte is visiting the university library and has made an appointment with the information specialist for nursing. She has decided on a broad topic, but wants her librarian's help to develop her search.

CHARLOTTE   Thanks for seeing me today.

LIBRARIAN (ANNA) Thank you for sending me your topic of interest, did you manage to refine it further with some of the techniques I suggested?

CHARLOTTE   Yes I tried the eyeball switch, because I read a report by the National Institute of Health Research (2019) that taking blood pressure medicine at night might help reduce cardio-vascular events and death. I wondered whether apart from this one recent study, there was any further evidence to support recommending a change in practice so that I would be able to advise patients in the future.

ANNA   So your question is. . .?

CHARLOTTE   I used PICO to formulate it: 'Is there evidence to suggest that taking antihypertensive medication at night (I) compared with taking it in the morning (C) reduces the incidence of cardiovascular events (O) in patients with high blood pressure (P)'.

ANNA   That sounds very good. Have you worked out your search terms and considered synonyms?

CHARLOTTE   Yes, I found 'antihypertensive agents' was an alternative term to medication on MEDLINE and 'medications' and 'drugs' are commonly used on CINAHL

ANNA   Good. Would 'evening doses' be a useful term as well as 'night-time medication'?

CHARLOTTE   It might and obviously I'll use 'hypertension' as well as 'high blood pressure'.

Charlotte and Anna try the search terms on MEDLINE and CINAHL, but do not find many hits. Anna suggests Charlotte reduce the number of terms she is trying to combine to see whether she is more successful. Charlotte tries again without combining her terms for the medications and night time with 'stroke' or synonyms for cardiovascular events and finds some interesting articles. Anna suggests that as the research Charlotte read about was very recent it may well be the first study of its kind and as such Charlotte may be better off readjusting her question.

Activity 6.2
Identify your topic of interest and formulate a question. Decide which databases appear most suitable for your area of interest. Work out your search terms and synonyms and conduct your initial search.

Did you find too many hits (you are overwhelmed), too few (you are frustrated with it) or just the right number to trawl through to decide whether they are useful?

Depending on your answer to the last question (and it would be unlikely to get it right first time) how can you refine your search? You might try changing your search terms, trying a different database, or using some of the search limits (e.g. date range, country, language). Think carefully about the Boolean operators AND, OR and NOT as well. Finding the best sources of evidence takes practice.

Conclusion

- Identify your topic.
- Formulate your question.
- Identify your search terms and synonyms.
- Identify the most relevant databases for your question.
- Conduct your search.
- Look at the type and number of hits you achieve and evaluate whether you need to refine your search.
- Re-run your search until you are finding suitable studies.

Once you have found a number of relevant studies you will be ready to begin to critically appraise them.

References

Farina, N., Llewellyn, D., Isaac, M.G.E.K.N. and Tabet, N. (2017) Vitamin E for Alzheimer's dementia and mild cognitive impairment. *Cochrane Database of Systematic Reviews*, (**4**), CD002854.

National Institute of Health Research (2019) Taking blood pressure medications at night seems best. https://discover.dc.nihr.ac.uk/content/signal-000851/taking-blood-pressure-medications-at-night-seems-best (accessed 16 January 2020).

For further resources for this chapter visit the companion website at
www.wiley.com/go/glasper/nursingdissertation2e

Chapter 7 What is grey literature and where can it be found?

Diane Carpenter[1] and Alan Glasper[2]
[1]*University of Plymouth, UK*
[2]*University of Southampton, UK*

Scenario

All the students have been asked by their academic supervisors to ensure that all aspects of grey literature have been explored and reflected in their review of the literature. Sue and Alisha are not at all clear how to identify 'grey literature' and they are concerned that they may miss a vital component to their literature searches.

All students completing evidence-based practice assignment or projects need to understand how to evaluate any grey literature pertinent to their field of study. The internet is now the largest source for the identification of grey literature.

What is 'grey literature'?

Firstly, grey literature is not grey! It comes in a variety of colours and sizes, some good, some bad and some just ugly. Grey literature is mainly composed of any literature that is not formally published in usual publishing formats such as textbooks or journal articles. Even Wikipedia is grey literature!

The term 'grey literature' refers primarily to scholarly papers, reports or other documents produced and published by, for example, Strategic Health Authorities, NHS Trusts, governmental agencies, universities and other

This chapter is based on an earlier chapter by Alan Glasper and Colin Rees.

How to Write Your Nursing Dissertation, Second Edition.
Edited by Alan Glasper and Diane Carpenter.
© 2021 John Wiley & Sons Ltd. Published 2021 by John Wiley & Sons Ltd.
Companion website: www.wiley.com/go/glasper/nursingdissertation2e

groups such as the Nursing and Midwifery Council (NMC) or the Care Quality Commission (CQC). Additionally, the royal colleges such as the Royal College of Nursing contain vast amounts of useful information as do a range of healthcare charities such as Age Concern.

These publications are not produced commercially, as in textbooks or journals, by well-known publishers and will therefore not have an ISBN (International Standard Book Number) or similar indexing. Although the internet has made a huge difference to how grey literature is sourced, many of these documents can be difficult to obtain. For example, many PhD theses still have to be borrowed from individual university libraries although many are available online. Significant contributions to the body of grey literature are translations from foreign language published papers.

Importantly, Alberani *et al.* (1990) have explored the importance of grey literature as a means of primary but non-conventionally published communication. It is important to stress that these bodies of literature, which are often original and of recent origin, cannot always be found easily through conventional channels.

Where can I find grey literature?

There are many websites that can help in locating and exploring the useful body of information contained in grey literature. Importantly, the World Wide Web has become the primary portal for sourcing grey literature in the twenty-first century.

The Healthcare Management Information Consortium (HMIC) database (Ovid) contains records from the Library and Information Services department of the Department of Health in England and the King's Fund Information and Library Service. These combined databases are considered to be a good source of grey literature on topics such as health and community care management, organisational development, inequalities in health, user involvement, and race and health.

DH Data is the database of the Department of Health's Library and Information Services and contains in excess of 174 000 records relating to health and social care management information. Coverage includes official publications, journal articles and grey literature on health service policy, management and administration, with an emphasis on the British National Health Service; the quality of health services including hospitals, nursing, primary care and public health; the planning, design, construction and maintenance of health service buildings; occupational health; control and regulation of medicines; medical equipment and supplies; and social care and personal social services. It includes all Department of Health publications, including circulars and press releases. The majority of records are from

1983 onwards, although coverage of departmental material dates back to 1919. Over one-quarter of the records have abstracts.

The King's Fund is an independent health charity that works to develop and improve management of health and social care services. The King's Fund Information and Library Service database holds records of the material in the library of the King's Fund Information and Library Service. The database contains over 70 000 records (1979 to date).

This Health Management and Policy Database from HMIC is an invaluable source of information for healthcare administrators and managers.

Important websites

A list of useful websites can be found on the companion site for this book. Go to www.wiley.com/go/glasper/nursingdissertation2e to find out more.

What about Google scholar?

> **Scenario**
>
> Charlotte has been asked by one of her fellow students if Google Scholar can be used as a shortcut to finding published and unpublished papers.

Jasco (2008) has highlighted the pros and cons of using Google Scholar to conduct a comprehensive literature search. Although Google Scholar is essentially a citation index – in other words papers have to be cited by other authors before they appear on the site – it is a very useful resource for healthcare students to use. Despite the weaknesses, Google Scholar enables users to search specifically for a wide range of scholarly literature.

References

Alberani, V., Pietrangeli, P. and Mazza, M.R. (1990) The use of grey literature in health sciences: a preliminary survey. *Bulletin of the Medical Library Association*, **78** (4), 358–362.

Jacso, P. (2008) The pros and cons of computing the h-index using Google Scholar. *Online Information Review*, **32** (3), 437–452.

For further resources for this chapter visit the companion website at
 www.wiley.com/go/glasper/nursingdissertation2e

Chapter 8 Harvard or Vancouver: getting it right all the time

Diane Carpenter[1] and Alan Glasper[2]
[1]*University of Plymouth, UK*
[2]*University of Southampton, UK*

Scenario

All the students have been instructed by their university faculty office to use the Harvard reference system. They have been informed that reference errors carry a 10% marking penalty. Sue, who is conscious of her lower grades as a diploma student, always found referencing difficult but she does not want to lose marks at this stage and thus jeopardise her eventual honours classification. Similarly Alisha struggles with reference techniques and often finds it difficult to get it right.

An important aspect of your project assignment is referencing the authors you have used throughout your work. This is part of academic work, where you are expected to provide evidence or support for the major statements you make and to the arguments you include in the dissertation/project. They are also required to avoid plagiarism, in that the words and ideas of others must be acknowledged in your work and must not be presented as if they are your own ideas. It is worth making the distinction between 'references', which includes all the authors whose work you have mentioned or 'referred' to in your dissertation, and 'bibliography', which includes work you may have read and found useful background work but is not directly referred to in your work. Many institutions do not require bibliographies, as there is no real evidence you have read them and so they may not be relevant.

This chapter is based on an earlier chapter by Alan Glasper and Colin Rees.

How to Write Your Nursing Dissertation, Second Edition.
Edited by Alan Glasper and Diane Carpenter.
© 2021 John Wiley & Sons Ltd. Published 2021 by John Wiley & Sons Ltd.
Companion website: www.wiley.com/go/glasper/nursingdissertation2e

References should be key to the topic and, as far as possible, be recent and not randomly sourced from Google Scholar. The way you show whose work you have included can take a number of different forms. The aim of this chapter is to consider the basic principles of referencing and illustrate the key features of the Vancouver and Harvard methods, two of the main referencing systems.

Referencing is an aspect of academic work that many people have found not difficult but irksome, as it is often responsible for some negative feedback comments on assignments. Yet by following some basic principles it is possible to avoid losing 'easy marks'.

Scenario

The students often meet in the coffee room and Sue asks Sam if he has problems with referencing as, no matter how much she tries, she always seems to lose marks and get comments about the standard of her referencing. Sam agrees it is something that has frequently frustrated him. They both decide to avoid losing important marks in their dissertations by having a session together to improve their referencing skills. Charlotte also finds this difficult, although her friend Alisha is quite happy with how to present references in her written work.

The form of referencing you use should be the one 'approved' by your institution. This will be stated in your course or programme handbook. As there are variations in the two systems we describe, it is recommended that you use both the system and variation suggested by your institution. This may require you to 'translate' some references that you might encounter into your 'approved' system.

Referencing systems relate to how you indicate a source of your reading in two parts of your work or dissertation: (i) in the body of your work and (ii) in the list of references at the end of your work. While the list is not usually included in your word count, those in the body are, so it is important to take this into account where you want to remain inside the word limit for your work.

Vancouver system

This system is not frequently used in UK universities but is frequently found in medical journals, so it is worth knowing how it works. It uses a number system for each source instead of using the name of the author or authors of a publication. It takes its name from a meeting of medical journal editors in Vancouver, Canada, in 1978. The problem for journals is how to make best use of space, so it was decided that those publishing in medical journals should allocate a number to each reference in turn and then list them in number order at the end. This would also help the flow of the article for the reader. The names of the journals were also abbreviated in the reference list to save more space. The numbers in the main body of a work are placed in brackets as close as possible to the statement it refers to, such as 'this has been shown in the work by Harrow [1] who found that. . ..' This is useful for students, as it is easy to type a number in brackets. Each time the same work is mentioned the original number is used again, so in the example above the work by Harrow would be [1] each time it was used. Where there are several authors you want to mention in relation to one point and they have already mentioned, if they are in order you can indicate this as follows: 'several authors have been seen to favour this method of assessment [3–6, 8, 10].'

Where you need to use a page number, this can be shown as follows, 'according to Harrow [1 p.6]. . ..' In journals the author number is also used in a more elaborate way by inserting a 'superscript' number, that is above the line, as in 'this has been shown in the work by Harrow[1] who found. . ..' Page numbers are then shown like this: 'according to Harrow[1(p.6)]. . ..' Table 8.1 shows some of the main features of the system. A number of versions are used, so always check which you are encouraged to use.

Harvard system

This has been in use a great deal longer than the Vancouver system and is adopted as the recommended style by many universities and most nursing journals. There are a number of variations of this too, so care has to be taken to always follow the version approved by your institution. Instead of numbers

Table 8.1 The Vancouver system.

Source to be used	How it would look in the references section
Book	1. Kent C. *Superbugs and Their Impact on Healthcare*. 3rd ed. Cardiff: Kimberly Press; 2012.
Chapter in a book	2. Parker P. The role of the nurse in supporting patients with arachnophobia. In: Allen B (ed.) *Fast Acting Treatments for Phobias and Anxiety States*. 3rd ed. Oxford: University Press; 2012, p.32–44.
Journal	3. Wayne B, Grayson D. Evidence-based practice and larvae therapy in wound care. *BJN* 2012;34(5):25–29.
Web-based reference	4. Prince D. Wonder and amazement; the lived experience of women caring for a child with chronic illness. *Qual Res Nurs* 2012. (accessed 29/11/2012)

Each reference is preceded by a number indicating its numeric sequence within the body of the work. This list assumes that the examples above appeared in sequence.

this uses the authors name and year of publication as the main identifiers in the main body of work. In the reference section the references are presented in alphabetical order and are not numbered or listed in the order in which they appear in the main body. Journal names are used in full. In the body of the work, the author's name and year are used in a number of different ways.

- As the subject of the sentence:
  'In the study by Johns (2012) it was shown that. . .'
  'Both Michael (2011) and Johns (2012) agree that. . .'
- Where the author provides the idea for the statement:
  'However, several authors have disagreed with this method (Michael 2011; Johns 2012).'

In the last example both the author's name and year of publication are in parentheses as they indicate the source of the information or point.

Where there are several authors of a single reference it is usual, if there are three or more names, to just use the first name in the body of your work followed by '*et al.*' and the year, where '*et al*' from the Latin means 'with others'. (Note that the use of Latin phrases in literature referencing is currently being debated.)

For example, 'Owen *et al.* (2011) found several examples. . .'. In the references section all the names are usually shown. However, as it has become increasingly popular for a large number of authors to be involved in publishing a single article, some referencing systems suggest that if there are six or more authors, list the first three followed by '*et al.*'.

There are some examples that need explanation, such as where an author is mentioned by a further author and you want to use the first author's point, and the following example explains this: 'Werther (2009) cited in Hauxwell (2011) believed that. . .'. In this example, only Hauxwell would appear in the reference section, as you have not read Werther's original work and the rule of referencing is that it is where you have read the work that must be indicated to the reader. This also applies to the Vancouver system.

The second difficulty often encountered is where the work is related to the author of a chapter in a book edited by someone else. In the main body you use the author's name and year the edited book was published as usual but in the references section it is shown as indicated in Table 8.2.

Notice that book titles and journal names are in italics and, unlike the Vancouver system, the title of the journal appears in full. The abbreviation for edition is 'edn.', unlike the Vancouver system that uses 'ed.' for both editor and edition depending on the context. You only need to show the edition number for second and subsequent editions; a first edition is not indicated.

Table 8.2 The Harvard system.

Source to be used	How it would look in the references section
Book	Kent, C. (2012) *Superbugs and Their Impact on Healthcare*, 3rd edn. Cardiff: Kimberly Press.
Chapter in a book	Parker, P. (2012) The role of the nurse in supporting patients with arachnophobia. In: Allen, B. (ed.) *Speedy Treatments for Phobias and Anxiety States*. Cardiff: Kimberly Press.
Journal	Wayne, B. and Grayson, D. (2012) The advantages of larvae therapy in wound care. *British Journal of Nursing* **34** (5), 25–29.
Web-based reference	Prince, D. (2012) Wonder and amazement: the lived experience of women caring for a child with chronic illness. *Qualitative Research in Nursing.* http://www. qualitativeresearchinnursing.oxfordjournals.com/contents/ pdf/6943-312-3-42.pdf (accessed 29/11/2012).

NB: This is not how they would appear in the references section as they would be listed in alphabetical order.

Both approaches to referencing illustrated in this chapter follow a similar goal of providing a systematic and consistent approach to listing the elements of a source of evidence. These will allow the reader to locate the information you used in your dissertation. Although similar elements are included, the order of the elements and the amount of detail does vary, so it is important not to confuse them and combine elements from both systems.

Use of computer referencing packages

There are a number of computer packages, such as EndNote, that can be purchased or obtained through your institution that will help put your references in order. These will allow you to enter the details for a reference and then provide it in a number of different formats. As always, the advice is that you should ensure that the result conforms with the system approved by your institution.

You will use many references in the course of developing your dissertation/ project. One of the best tips is to start the references section when you start writing your first draft. The first time you include a reference in the draft, start your reference section either in a separate file or by pressing enter ten times, putting the heading 'References' and then writing the reference in full in the approved system. Each new reference should be added in the appropriate place. Once the dissertation is complete, the reference section will also be complete and will just need to be checked if any references have been added or deleted at any stage without the reference section being adjusted.

Conclusion

As the standard of your referencing says something about your attention to detail and your academic standard, it is worth ensuring that your referencing skills are high. This chapter should have increased your understanding of the two main systems and how to complete appropriate references for a range of sources.

For further resources for this chapter visit the companion website at
   www.wiley.com/go/glasper/nursingdissertation2e

Chapter 9 Posing an evidence-based practice question: using the PICO and SPICE models

Alan Glasper[1] and Diane Carpenter[2]
[1]University of Southampton, UK
[2]University of Plymouth, UK

Scenario

Sam has selected a likely topic for his dissertation. He wants to explore the lived experiences of families with a child with a chronic illness but wants to ensure that it is suitable for a dissertation subject. He talks to Sue about her choice, which is the use of larvae therapy for wound healing in older women with varicose leg ulcers. During a class discussion Sue has been struggling with framing her question using the PICO or SPICE model. Their lecturers have been explicit in the need to formulate an answerable question using one of these models. They have also been instructed to pose their evidence-based practice question at the conclusion of their dissertation introductory chapter before writing the literature search chapter. Although Charlotte and Alisha are not undertaking a full dissertation, both have to search the evidence-based literature as part of their project and assignment. Their lecturers have advised them to use a model such as PICO or SPICE. This is because it is important to stress that the creation of a precise and answerable question will facilitate a more efficient literature search and the eventual retrieval of suitable published papers. After a full interrogation and critical appraisal of these papers an individual will be able to come to a conclusion as to whether the answer to the question will potentially allow a change in practice. There are a number of models designed to help in the formulation of an answerable question. Only the PICO and SPICE models are considered here.

This chapter is based on an earlier chapter by Alan Glasper and Colin Rees.

How to Write Your Nursing Dissertation, Second Edition.
Edited by Alan Glasper and Diane Carpenter.
© 2021 John Wiley & Sons Ltd. Published 2021 by John Wiley & Sons Ltd.
Companion website: www.wiley.com/go/glasper/nursingdissertation2e

What is the PICO model?

Straus *et al.* (2005) outlined the PICO model of formulating a focused and answerable question. There are four elements to the posing of a PICO question. These four common features of the PICO format are helpful in allowing healthcare practitioners to carefully consider the questions they wish the literature they interrogate to answer. Melnyk and Fineout-Overholt (2005) believe that each aspect of the PICO format should be considered in depth to generate a clearly articulated question. The four elements are:

P   Population
I   Intervention
C   Comparison
O   Outcome.

Booth (2006) outlines each element of the PICO model as follows.

Population
The recipients or potential beneficiaries of a service or intervention. The population can be patients or clients with, for example:

- a disease or condition (patients with gastrointestinal disease);
- a stage of disease (patients with advanced Crohn's disease);
- a specific gender (women with postnatal depression);
- age group (children with Crohn's disease);
- socioeconomic group (semi-skilled and unskilled manual workers with alcohol-related disease);
- healthcare setting (mental healthcare patients attending an outpatient department).

Intervention
The service or planned action that is being delivered to the population. This could be one of a number of interventions, for example:

- a type of drug therapy for renal disease, surgical procedures used in renal disease, types of radiotherapy used in treating malignancies, and so on;
- a level of intervention, for example the frequency of administration of a particular medication or the dosage of a particular drug or radiotherapy treatment;
- the stage of intervention, for example possibly expressed as prevention, secondary or advanced;
- the delivery of an intervention, for example by intravenous infusion or by self-medication.

Comparison

An alternative service or action that may or may not achieve similar outcomes. For example, the use of peritoneal dialysis as a comparison with haemodialysis or the use of antibiotic drug A compared with antibiotic drug B. In some cases the comparison may be the usual named interventions or no intervention. Some questions are formulated without a comparison if the intention is to understand the effect of a specific intervention on the outcome for a designated population.

Outcomes

The ways in which the service or action can be measured to establish whether or not it has had a desired effect. This can be expressed as what happened to the population being studied as a direct result of the intervention. This can be articulated in a number of ways.

- It might be specifically patient oriented, as in an improvement in quality of life, a reduction in the severity of their symptoms, or a reduction in adverse events such as drug errors. However, these should be expressed in measurable ways such as 'lower pain scores', 'fewer episodes of nausea and vomiting', anything that shows there has been a clear and measurable difference as a result of the intervention.
- It might also be organisation orientated, such as cost-effectiveness, fewer days in hospital, or a reduction in the number of personal injury claims or complaints by patients.

In this way, Huang *et al.* (2006) have suggested that the use of the mnemonic PICO helps practitioners to more precisely pose a clinically related question in trying to answer a perceived clinical problem. Additionally, using the PICO framework will result in improved literature search strategies using the words in the PICO statement as the key search terms in the databases. This will generate more accurate results that are more likely to locate data-driven papers that when subjected to critical appraisal will help to provide support or rejection of the proposed intervention.

Examples of PICO formulated questions

Tip

This section is designed to allow you an opportunity to examine a range of questions that might help you consider the formulation of your own dissertation question and search strategy key words.

Chapter 9

PICO question example 1 (a humorous example)

In 1999, the 23rd Annual Report of the Home Accident Surveillance System (http://docplayer.net/7094813-Hass-23rd-annual-report-welcome.html) estimated that 3695 accidents in the UK involved trousers. Although the annual report does not specify what type of injury, it could be zipper related or simply caused by falling whilst removing them. First and crucially in the process of undertaking an evidence-based practice enquiry is to formulate an answerable question. Were students seriously looking to address the accident rate caused by trousers, a PICO question might be formulated as follows.

Population	Trouser-wearing men over 30 years of age.
Intervention	Replacing trousers with kilts.
Comparison	None, or perhaps togas (why not, as the toga movie, once the oldest of the Hollywood movie genres, is suddenly back in fashion).
Outcome	A reduction in the number of trouser-related injuries.

This could then be written thus: For trouser-wearing men over 30 years of age, does replacing trousers with kilts compared with togas reduce the number of trouser-related injuries?

PICO question example 2 (more serious)

It is very important when using PICO to formulate focused and answerable questions, *not* for example 'Are febrile convulsions in babies dangerous?' In this example there is no intervention (I), comparison (C), or outcome (O) measure. The answer to such a question may simply be 'yes' and so result in a very short dissertation!

Ask specific, focused and answerable questions, for example 'Does a febrile convulsion in a nine-month-old infant increase the likelihood that they develop convulsions in later life?' However, this can go even further and provide a well-structured dissertation if you think about best practice and the interventions that may help reduce the rate of convulsions. So, you may improve on this by considering an intervention and comparison as follows.

Population	Infants under one year of age who have suffered from a febrile convulsion.
Intervention	Treatment following UK National Institute for Health and Care Excellence (NICE) guidelines (http://www.nice.org.uk/cg047).
Comparison	The use of antipyretic medication.
Outcome	A reduction in the number of convulsions in later life.

PICO question example 3
Is acupuncture effective in improving recovery from stroke?

Population	Men over 60 years of age who have suffered a stoke.
Intervention	Acupuncture: duration of treatment, frequency and so on.
Comparison	Standard stoke rehabilitation programmes.
Outcome	Higher stroke recovery rate measured in time, and scale to measure level of mobility.

PICO question example 4
Is the use of exercise more efficient than antidepressants for treating depression in women over 40 years of age?

Population	Women suffering from depression: severity, from a particular socioeconomic group, from a specific healthcare setting?
Intervention	Exercise: what type (e.g. running), how strenuous, how often (e.g. twice daily)?
Comparison	Antidepressant medication: type, dose, frequency and duration?
Outcome	Lower level of depression as measured by a depression scale.

PICO question example 5
Does the use of antibiotics for middle ear infection in children under five years of age reduce the incidence of mastoiditis?

Population	Preschool children with acute otitis media: socioeconomic factors or households with ambient tobacco residue?
Intervention	Antibiotics: which antibiotic, what dose, how frequent, which method of administration?
Comparison	No intervention.
Outcome	Number of subsequent episodes of mastoiditis (cost-effectiveness?).

PICO question example 6 (a biblical example)
In Chapter 3 we cited the first recorded clinical trial, which features in the Old Testament and which clearly shows an allocation of children to a dietary group, one group eating the royal foods of King Nebuchadnezzar, namely meat and wine, and the other group a vegetarian diet in the form of pulses with water only. The aim of this trial was to ascertain differences in 'countenance' (usually referring to appearance but especially related to the face and how it is perceived by onlookers).

Chapter 9

Population	Israeli children and Israeli children from the royal families (N = unknown). Inclusion criteria included blemish-free, wise, able to learn a language, and with an understanding of science (remember gender was not stated!).
Intervention	A new diet consisting of the King's meat (not stated but possibly lamb, chicken or maybe goat or even camel) and wine (this is not stipulated but was it red or white, what was the grape variety, was it grown on south-facing vineyards and, importantly, what percentage of alcohol did it contain and how much did they drink – was it more than 14 units per week?).
Comparison	Four children including Daniel who had a diet of pulses (not stated in the Old Testament but it may have been broad beans or perhaps fava beans) and water (not stated in the Old Testament but was it still or sparkling or just water from the well?).
Outcome	Countenance. (Is this a valid measure of health and how is it measured? Is there a 'countenance scale' to provide a numeric value?)

Many researchers find the PICO model appropriate for a whole range of clinical questions.

What is the SPICE model?

The SPICE model has been proposed by Booth and Brice (2004) and is a derivation of the PICO model. It was designed originally for use primarily by librarians to help to more clearly focus some types of literature search enquiry that did not always fit the PICO framework. The SPICE model framework has five components and is helpful for students who are not asking a clinically focused question. The mnemonic SPICE stands for:

Setting	Where and what is the context?
Perspective	For whom? Who are users/potential users of service?
Intervention	What is being done to them/for them?
Comparison	Compared with what? What are alternatives?
Evaluation	With what result and how will you measure whether the intervention will succeed?

Although the SPICE structure is similar to that of PICO, Booth (2009) points out that by separating the traditional medical-type population aspect of the

PICO model into, firstly, a setting and, secondly, a perspective this enables SPICE to be used for posing non-medical type questions, in other words more of a social scientific approach. Similarly, by substituting the term 'outcome' with the term 'evaluation' the SPICE model of posing a question facilitates other elements of research which are broader and incorporate concepts such as outputs or impacts.

SPICE question example 1

The first example is from the Belgian Health Care Knowledge Centre (KCE). This is a semi-governmental institution which analyses healthcare data from various research studies with the aim of improving evidence-based practice.

What is the impact of an increase in the level of cost sharing on access to health services for the chronically ill in European countries?

Setting	(A selection of) European countries.
Perspective	Chronically ill patients.
Intervention	Increased cost sharing (from among the European Community).
Comparison	No increase in current funding arrangements.
Evaluation	Access to health services.

Activity 9.1

Access the Belgian Health Care Knowledge Centre (KCE) (https://www.inahta.org/members/kce/) and investigate the various research questions hosted there using the SPICE model.

SPICE question example 2

How does it feel to wait for your relative (child, spouse/partner or parent) to return to the ward after emergency surgery and await the results?

Setting	Hospital surgical wards.
Perspective	Relatives of patients requiring emergency surgery.
Intervention	Dedicated waiting area with refreshments and tangible levels of distraction, such as flat screen televisions or contemporary topical magazines.
Comparison	No special area or levels of distraction.
Evaluation	By questionnaire given to relative when leaving the hospital or on return home.

Chapter 9

Scenario

All the students now understand how to pose an answerable question and how this links to their search strategy for their literature reviews. They also have two clear ways in which they can structure their question depending on the nature of their topic area.

Activity 9.2

- Go the book website at www.wiley.com/go/glasper/nursingdissertation2e and download the PICO and SPICE mnemonic proformas.
- Practice writing answerable questions in your learning group.

References

Booth, A. (2006) Clear and present questions: formulating questions for evidence based practice. *Library Hi Tech*, **24** (3), 355–368. DOI: 10.1108/07378830610692127.

Booth, A. (2009) A bridge too far? Stepping stones for evidence-based practice in an academic context. *New Review of Academic Librarianship*, **15**, 3–34.

Booth, A. and Brice, A. (2004) *Formulating Answerable Questions*. Evidence Based Practice: *An Information Professional's Handbook*. Facet, London.

Huang, X., Lin, J. and Demner-Fushman, D. (2006) Evaluation of PICO as a knowledge representation for clinical questions. AMIA Annual Symposium Proceedings, pp. 359–363.

Melnyk, B.M. and Fineout-Overholt, E. (2005) Evidence-Based Practice in Nursing and Health Care. A Guide to Best Practice, p. 29. Lippincott Williams & Wilkins, Philadelphia.

Straus, S.E., Richardson, W.S., Glasziou, P. and Haynes, R.B. (2005) Evidence-Based Medicine: How to Practice and Teach EBM, 3rd edn, p. 257. Churchill Livingstone Elsevier, London.

For further resources for this chapter visit the companion website at

www.wiley.com/go/glasper/nursingdissertation2e

Section 3 **Developing your healthcare/ evidence-based practice dissertation**

The students are learning to use the bibliographical databases to kick-start their search for appropriate literature to underpin their work. They have been given access to a complete sample dissertation (which is part of this book's electronic resource) which allows them to see first-hand how the architecture of a dissertation is constructed. All are conscious of how they must use their time wisely to ensure that they meet their deadlines.

Chapter 10 **Managing your time wisely**

Diane Carpenter[1] and Alan Glasper[2]
[1]*University of Plymouth, UK*
[2]*University of Southampton, UK*

Scenario

All the students have got mixed feelings about the task ahead of them. On the one hand they are excited about exploring a topic and learning something new through it. They are also eager to gain the best mark possible for their work. This is especially so for Sue and Charlotte where the marks received count towards the classification of their degrees. However, the size of the evidence-based practice healthcare dissertation/final project or evidence-informed decision-making assignment is worrying them, as are the demands it will make on their time. Sue keeps thinking of her family and trying to fit things in. Sam is thinking about his job and the other interests he has in life. They both share their concerns and agree it is knowing how to start the work and not let life events take over from the work on the dissertation while at the same time 'having a life!' Sue has her family, as well as her work, and there are many events that will occur during the time of the dissertation that will be difficult to ignore. Sam also has family obligations and tries to regularly look after his health through sessions at the gym and keep friendship ties going. Charlotte and Alisha both have busy social lives and are nervous about leaving the work until the last minute.

These reactions to the work ahead are very typical of students starting an evidence-based practice healthcare dissertation/final project or evidence-informed decision-making assignment. Although this kind of activity is often the last piece of work for a programme of study, it is often seen as an

This chapter is based on an earlier chapter by Alan Glasper and Colin Rees.

How to Write Your Nursing Dissertation, Second Edition.
Edited by Alan Glasper and Diane Carpenter.
© 2021 John Wiley & Sons Ltd. Published 2021 by John Wiley & Sons Ltd.
Companion website: www.wiley.com/go/glasper/nursingdissertation2e

almost impossible task because of the work involved, and this will need to be accommodated into an already busy and cramped life. Unless these problems can be seen in context and some action plans developed, the experience of undertaking an evidence-based practice healthcare dissertation/final project or evidence-informed decision-making assignment is not going to be a happy one. What is the answer to this problem?

The aim of this chapter is to consider how you might improve time management so that the demands of this forthcoming work can be integrated with other demands in your life. Some key principles will be suggested that will make this easier to achieve.

There are a number of things that must happen at the start of this period. Firstly, the activity of undertaking the work must be seen as an opportunity and not a threat. Secondly, the activity needs to be divided into various stages that can then be allocated a time frame that will make the whole job seem manageable. Thirdly, you need to seize control of your time and activities so that you can pace the work to reach the deadline with the minimum of extra stress in your life. So, we are talking about a frame of mind or attitude needed to tackle a dissertation, and then a plan of action that will match a timetable.

An evidence-based practice healthcare dissertation/final project or evidence-informed decision-making assignment as a frame of mind

Complex work such as a dissertation will take over your life; it will certainly take over your living space. You may find yourself waking up thinking about it, and it may delay you getting to sleep. This may seem like a nightmare but it does not have to be. The evidence-based practice healthcare dissertation/final project or evidence-informed decision-making assignment is something that shows you can work on your own, applying all the skills you have learnt through your programme of study. Often they focus on a clinical or professional problem and when complete they represent your contribution to the professional body of knowledge. If you see it as a growing friend and accept that it will only be in your life for a relatively short period, until the submission date, then it will become more manageable. Your first task is to make a friend of your evidence-based practice healthcare dissertation/final project or evidence-informed decision-making assignment and welcome it into your life.

The second task is to make a space for it in your life. This means seeing it as something that will require you to give it time and provide it with food and nurture so that it will grow in size and, finally, 'move away from home' – your home – once the work is complete and submitted to the university for marking. Northedge (2005) suggests you need to become skilled in creating time

---

Scenario

One of Sam's friends who recently completed a master's dissertation, towards the end of this work regularly set his wake-up alarm on his iPhone to give him two extra study hours before going to work several times a week. Although he became somewhat temporally fixated, other students not so inclined have been known take a month's holiday on a Greek island and take their notebook computers and write up the work in one hit. Not recommended, but whatever works for you!

The former is usually safer than the latter.

---

in which it can sit, either by stopping or reducing an alternative activity, or gaining more time in the week when it is possible to focus on your work. For many people it may simply be a better use of scheduled time and putting some things on hold for the duration of the evidence-based practice health-care dissertation/final project or evidence-informed decision-making assignment. The example of Sam's friend, however, shows it is possible to create time.

To help you schedule your time, it is useful to divide the whole process into a number of sections composed of a number of activities. This allows you to put a time against each activity and fit it into a space that will allow you to complete it. Together these activities will allow you to complete each section of the work to arrive at the final deadline. If this is to work smoothly, good time management, as Cottrell (2008) observes is absolutely essential. This is because you must take control of the work, as there will be the minimum of guidance from others. Unlike regular module attendance, there will probably be very few timetabled sessions to help you pace your written work.

The whole evidence-based practice healthcare dissertation/final project or evidence-informed decision-making assignment can be seen as having a beginning, a middle, and an end. Surprisingly, the place to start is the end. This is where you will conclude your work by answering the aim you decided on at the very beginning of the journey. Now, put the submission date minus two weeks as the finishing point. This will give you a margin of two weeks to get it all finished and submitted either electronically or as a hard-bound paper copy depending on the university. Then take a further two weeks off for the final editing of the sections and making sure there is consistency in things like the headings you have used, ensuring that all tables or other 'inserts' are correctly numbered and that the contents page is complete with the right numbers against each element. The abstract and acknowledgements may also need to be completed in this phase. You might find it helpful to use a time chart such as a Gantt chart (see Chapter 1).

Chapter 10

Before your end section, you will need a 'middle' that will contain the bulk of your work. This is often in the form of a review of the literature where you critically examine all the evidence in the form of published papers you have collected. For this section you will need to do three things:

1. source appropriate literature;
2. read and extract appropriate points from the literature you have sourced;
3. write rough drafts of the section having decided what goes where and synthesising the material with your own 'voice' so that it leads to a clear conclusion.

The best advice is not to perform these in sequence as separate activities but to do them at the same time. You will find it a great advantage to your growing understanding of the topic and your own evidence-based practice healthcare dissertation/final project or evidence-informed decision-making assignment if, when you read through your articles, you write some preliminary thoughts in the form of notes for yourself about what other work they may link to, so that this will make the synthesis of the work easier. You may wish to review the sample guidelines detailed in Chapter 2 before proceeding further.

Now the beginning: this is where you will develop the rationale and background for your choice of topic once it has been decided. The most important tip at this point is to avoid developing your aim until you are quite sure there is accessible information available to build up your evidence-based practice healthcare dissertation/final project or evidence-informed decision-making assignment. It is this beginning section that can be the most difficult up to the point that you decide on the topic that has the appropriate amount of literature to sustain it. This also needs a start time to it and a cut-off point where you start work on the middle section.

Each of the three broad sections will contain the same themes such that the whole evidence-based practice healthcare dissertation/final project or evidence-informed decision-making assignment 'hangs together' and develops right the way from beginning to end and flows back again. This means that the beginning may change slightly over time as themes may merge or get taken out. Whatever themes are in one section must appear in the other sections, so when working on one section you may be able to add some notes for yourself in your draft of earlier or later sections. Always remember any section should always be seen as 80% complete. You may go back and make changes depending on what you encounter or decide later down the road to writing your dissertation/project/assignment.

You should now have in your mind three broad sections that all exist at the same time as you will work across these sections at the same time. Although you will be mainly focusing on one section when you work on your dissertation/project/dissertation, you may need to add something, even if only a note to yourself in brackets, at the same time in one of the other sections.

In each section there are activities that have to be complete by the end of the process, so we can now produce your dissertation/project/assignment timetable. Allocate time for each of these activities, looking carefully at your calendar of events and making space for family and other occasions that need to be given time. Construct for yourself and your academic supervisor a work plan that looks something like Table 10.1 containing target dates for completion. Using the 'actions' in Table 10.1 as a guide, slot in the dates starting with the last one and working back to the present. If any of them look a little 'odd' or out of sync, then make some readjustments. Ensure realistic target dates and then share these with your academic supervisor so they can help you keep to time.

You should now find that you have cut the evidence-based practice healthcare dissertation/final project or evidence-informed decision-making assignment down to size by seeing it as a series of activities that need to be project managed against tasks to be completed within a timetable of dates. These dates should dovetail into a social diary.

Table 10.1 Example of a timetable for an evidence-based practice healthcare dissertation/final project or evidence-informed decision-making assignment.

Target date	Action
Deadline 1 (write as dates)	Select topic, check literature is there to support it. Start the written work diary to record progress and key decisions and 'to-do' list. Write draft rationale/background to the topic. Give the work a title in the form of a statement, and an aim that begins, 'the aim of this dissertation/project/assignment is to. . .'. Send this to your academic supervisor and arrange a meeting to discuss
Deadline 2	Write a plan to follow to search the literature including databases, using key words, and a time frame, plus inclusion and exclusion criteria. Search the literature following your plan, adjusting your plan or search as necessary. Keep track of the hits per database and how numbers of possible inclusions are reduced into those finally included in your literature critique. As the literature is gathered, quickly read, make notes, decide in which section to place it and how it will integrate with other work
Deadline 3	Write a search strategy and draft the early section of the review. Send this to your academic supervisor who will check your approach
Deadline 4	Complete the search of the literature section and compile a first draft of the review of the literature
Deadline 5	Complete sections following the literature review, e.g. change sections, recommendations
Deadline 6	Before moving into the final sections such as conclusions, read through the work to date and ensure you have a clear idea of the shape of the assignment and map out where it is going in the final sections

Chapter 10

(Continued)

Table 10.1 (Continued)

Target date	Action
Deadline 7	Complete first draft of the whole of the evidence-based practice healthcare dissertation/final project or evidence-informed decision-making assignment excluding sections before the introduction. Check that your conclusion matches your stated aim. Check all your references
Deadline 8	Complete sections before introduction, such as the abstract, acknowledgements and contents page, and check pages in work correspond with those in contents page. Check all tables and boxes have headings and titles and are listed in contents page following main sections under heading 'Tables/Boxes'
Deadline 9	Spend two weeks on editing, reading to make sense of everything. Check all headings are in a similar format, all references correct and listed. Check dissertation/project/ assignment guidelines and requirements against the work completed to ensure nothing is missing and everything has been considered. Final preparation for submission, such as any binding or checking method of electronic submission
Deadline 10	Submission date. Deliver the evidence-based practice healthcare dissertation/final project or evidence-informed decision-making assignment according to your plan. Celebrate!

Conclusion

There are a number of strategies you can employ in order to achieve the best use of your precious time. Planning is a key aspect of evidence-based practice healthcare dissertations/final projects or evidence-informed decision-making assignments and coordination of the activities that go to make up each part of the work. Get support from those around you and try to keep to a timetable that is realistic and gives you some balance in life. Try to allocate so many hours a week to work on the dissertation/project assignment and set a target of so many words per week or per 10 days. Record this in your written work diary and you will be surprised at how quickly the words mount up. Do not leave the writing until the very end as you will put yourself under too much stress and lose a lot of the good ideas you had as you went along. When you set yourself a weekly work schedule for your written work, try to add a little time or an extra session so that if something unexpected happens you can be flexible in the way you cope with it. All these will contribute to you feeling in control of the work, and will not leave you feeling stressed and exhausted. An evidence-based practice healthcare dissertation/final project or evidence-informed decision-making assignment is something that should be enjoyed but you need to give yourself time to achieve that.

Scenario

Following this advice, the students feel that many of their anxieties about finding time to undertake the work have reduced. It is a lot of work, but they have found that having a clearer picture of the activities and the need to keep pushing forward with it has made it manageable and achievable. They have also ensured that those around them know they are going to need support but that it is for a set period, after which things can return more to normal.

References

Cottrell, S. (2008) *The Study Skills Handbook*, 3rd edn. Palgrave Macmillan, Basingstoke, UK.

Northedge, A. (2005) *The Good Study Guide*, 2nd edn. Open University, Milton Keynes, UK.

For further resources for this chapter visit the companion website at
   www.wiley.com/go/glasper/nursingdissertation2e

Chapter 10

Chapter 11 **Developing your study skills**

Diane Carpenter[1], and Alan Glasper[2]
[1] *University of Plymouth, UK*
[2] *University of Southampton, UK*

Why do we need to consider study skills in this book? It is because at degree or foundation degree level and as part of your evidence-based practice healthcare dissertation/final project or evidence-informed decision-making assignment you will need to be an independent learner. There will be fewer people telling you what to do and less 'contact' time to get direction. The direction and major decisions come from you. This means you cannot leave it until it gradually becomes clear to you what is going on; you have to be in control of your own learning and be proactive. Without this kind of approach, you may suddenly find that the submission date is almost upon you and all you have are some quick notes you made so long ago that you find it difficult to understand what you originally wrote.

The evidence-based practice healthcare dissertation/final project or evidence-informed decision-making assignment is about bringing together a large number of skills at the right time so that there are no hold ups or 'dead time' while you are waiting for things to happen. As far as possible you should

---

Scenario

Sam and Alisha are concerned because both have been out of studying a little while and have forgotten all the things that make a course and an activity like writing an assignment easy. Sue has found she can confidently tackle certain parts of assignments like the background reading, which she quite enjoys, but gets a little unsure about what she is supposed to write. Charlotte has an identified learning difference and has problems with getting work finished on time. They all realise that what they need to do is consider their personal strengths and limitations when it comes to study skills.

This chapter is based on an earlier chapter by Alan Glasper and Colin Rees.

How to Write Your Nursing Dissertation, Second Edition.
Edited by Alan Glasper and Diane Carpenter.
© 2021 John Wiley & Sons Ltd. Published 2021 by John Wiley & Sons Ltd.
Companion website: www.wiley.com/go/glasper/nursingdissertation2e

try to carry out activities in parallel so that you can coordinate task that need to be completed at the same time.

The aim of this chapter is to consider some of the study skills that are appropriate to an evidence-based practice healthcare dissertation/final project or evidence-informed decision-making assignment. In reading this you will find you are already doing some of them, but you should find that there will be some new ideas that will help you get over some of the challenges to this written work, especially if you identify with similar issues to the scenario characters.

The essential skills for dissertations are those shown in Figure 11.1. They are essential as they move the whole activity forward and they must be of the right level to get you the best grade for your achievements. (NB: you should always aim to get the best classification for your undergraduate or postgraduate work.) The good thing about these activities is that they work together, and collectively make up the key feature of your dissertation/project/assignment. The diagram can be seen as a 'dynamic' model in that each of the corners of the triangle are in constant motion and working with the other parts of the triangle. Wherever you start you must take the other two into account.

One of the key areas in an evidence-based practice healthcare dissertation/final project or evidence-informed decision-making assignment is that of critical analysis. This is not an easy idea to convey and a number of chapters in this book are designed to help you develop this skill. It does not mean the skill to be critical but to be able to make judgements based on sound principles. At degree/foundation degree level it is showing that you can make balanced judgements and support your comments with reasoning and evidence from other authors to support your statements. This means exploring the statements made by authors as well as considering any assumptions that go with the statements and whether you feel the statements are reasonable and supported by evidence and other authors. Part of critical analysis is indicating to your reader not only what someone says but what you feel about what someone says.

Chapter 11

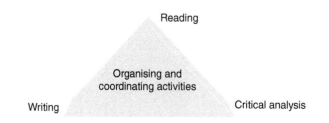

Figure 11.1 Model showing key skills areas in developing your written work.

What are they basically saying?	What do I think of this?

Figure 11.2 Critical analysis skills table.

To help you think about developing your skills in critical analysis, consider using a simple two-column table (Figure 11.2). The left-hand column of the table can be used to jot down notes on 'What are they basically saying?' The right-hand column can be used to write down notes on 'What do I think of this?', especially 'so what are the implications of this?' Then when reading an article or textbook fill in the columns and use this technique until you do not need the columns and you begin to automatically read things with these two questions in mind. This will develop your ability to start thinking critically. Make sure that for the right-hand side you think 'What are the positive things about this, and what are the possible limitations?'; that is, where they are appropriate to the point. Once you master this skill you can begin to contemplate using the sophisticated critiquing tools that are discussed in other chapters of this book.

Study skills are about how you study by being aware of what time of day suits you best for studying, how long to study at one time before you lose concentration, or if by changing your activity when this happens you can still continue to achieve something in that time slot.

Knowing yourself

Knowing when to seek the help of your friends and supervisor if you start to fall behind your work schedule or if you feel that things are getting on top of you is a valuable skill. These are indicators that you need to do things slightly differently. It is knowing who to approach and being clear in what it is you would like to change. Additionally, if you feel that you may have a learning difference, as with undergraduate student Charlotte, that is impacting on your ability to produce work of a good standard, you must approach your faculty learning support advisor as early as possible (see Chapter 26).

Both writing and reading are groups of activities that consist of a number of different elements.

Writing
- Notes for self
- Preliminary 'rough' drafts
- More formal work
- Final draft work

Reading
- Journal articles and recommended textbooks
- Reading your own notes

The first aspect of managing your reading is finding what to read. Completing your evidence-based practice healthcare dissertation/final project or evidence-informed decision-making assignment will depend on you finding relevant material to answer your research-based question/topic. One key skill is learning how to make fast and efficient use of databases and not to depend on search engines to do this for you. Chapter 6 explains this in detail. Importantly, databases contain work from peer-reviewed journals which are a better quality source of knowledge on subjects. To make best use of them check your timetable schedule for programmed sessions on searching databases that might be part of your module or arrange to attend a session that the university library might organise for students. One of the sections in your review of the literature will be details on your search strategy and you will need to keep track of the databases you use, the key search words, the time frame covered, and any specific inclusion and exclusion criteria that helped you focus down from a large number of hits to a manageable number to include in your literature review. A search details grid may help you keep track of this and some authors have developed search grids for this purpose (Rees, 2010). Chapter 6 gives more details of how to use quality databases.

When you find articles you also need to keep track of them, and you may wish to use folders with 'theme' labels to help keep together topic articles that go together.

Extracting information that might be used in your evidence-based practice healthcare dissertation/final project or evidence-informed decision-making assignment can also be managed in a grid. The purpose of a grid is to allow you to collect information together from different articles under the same column headings, so that you can compare and contrast information from different authors. You will find it an advantage to slot these into a grid so that they appear in year order with the most recent articles first. This has the additional advantage of enabling you to compare trends over time with the findings, sample composition or size, method of data collection and, of course, main findings and recommendations.

You will see examples of these when reviewing the literature articles; they will look like the grid shown in Figure 11.3. The headings used here are only suggestions and you can adapt the idea to match the theme headings that are relevant to your dissertation. (A sample of a commonly used grid is detailed in Chapter 17, and this grid is also appended to the companion website www. wiley.com/go/glasper/nursingdissertation2e.)

For the last column it is always useful to end with 'my comments', in which you include what you found particularly interesting or what may be a possible limitation. This then acts as a prompt for your critical analysis. The grid in Figure 11.3 is presented in 'portrait' format (running down the page) but you will find it a lot easier to reproduce in 'landscape' format (running across the page) so the columns are wider and can accommodate more text. Reducing the font size to something like 10 point or even 8 point will also increase how much detail you can include.

Many people find it useful to use highlighter pens to first identify possible information in hard copies of articles before transferring them to a grid. Highlighter pens can also be used to identify the common themes you have divided your review into, so green might highlight problems related to your topic and yellow possible solutions (Chapter 17 gives details of how to use highlighter pens). These make it easier to pick themes out, but also help in telling you at a glance if an article is more 'problem' focused or 'answer' focused. It is techniques like this that will allow you to see the bigger picture and make comments that will get you more marks than just being descriptive.

For reading it is important to become an active reader. This is different from reading a novel where you can just let the words flow over you as the images of the story emerge and take shape. Reading non-fiction is not like that. It is important to remain alive to the messages that a journal article or textbook contains. Here it is important to be continually asking questions or 'interrogating the text' in terms of the key messages it contains and the way it fits into what has already been read. One tip is to read the first sentence in

Author/ Year	Aim	Sample and size	Tool of data collection	Main findings	Recommendations	My comments

Figure 11.3 Example of a data extraction grid.

each paragraph as that is often the 'topic sentence' that contains the main point of the paragraph. Just scanning down the pages reading the first sentence can often help you to get a total picture very quickly. The same also applies to your drafts, where you can check if your work is flowing by reading the first sentence in every paragraph. There should be some kind of clear narrative when you read first lines. You may need to reconsider how you are presenting material if it does not flow.

Reading each article from your search may take you longer than you think; you can also quickly feel 'saturated' with the information and lose interest in an article, especially if it contains complex terms and statistics. Try not to be too ambitious in each 'reading session' you do. Set yourself either just one article or so much of an article, but transfer the information into a grid or make notes as you go along. This will mean you will not have to read the whole article again from the beginning but can read your grid or notes to catch up to where you left off. You will quickly find that the grid builds up and you begin to see the picture it contains based on the articles you have read. Always keep several copies of your papers so that you can have one in your handbag or briefcase which you can read on boats, buses trains and aeroplanes or during your lunch or coffee break.

Bringing all the activities together in a coordinated and meaningful way in a space given for your dissertation/project/assignment is important. This is a creative activity and one that you can be proud of the results. It should not be raced through with the aim to get it behind you as quickly as possible.

Being organised

Very few people have too much spare time on their hands, especially when working on a complex piece of written work. The issue is one of prioritising the many tasks you have to complete in the various phases of this work and formulating precisely where you should be spending your time so that you make best use of it. Things that might help are '*to-do*' lists that are weighted into those that must be done sooner than others, for example using a coding system of A, B and C, with As being done before Bs, and so on.

One important area of prioritising is related to the reading you will have to do. This applies especially when you are reviewing the literature, as there will be a lot to read in a short space of time when you are trying to gain a quick view of articles that will be of help to you. A simple system when you have downloaded or run off an article is to quick scan it, make an assessment of its value and then in the top left-hand corner above the title give it a 1–5 star rating, with the more potentially useful articles having the greater number of stars. Hence, very relevant up-to-date articles may get four or five stars, whilst an older article with only the odd good definition or point will get two or three stars. Sort your articles by star rating and make sure you read the high-star articles first. You will be wasting your time if you give equal weight to each article.

A big part of being a successful student is being very organised with the amount of work you have to cope with. Some of this will relate to clearly seeing how much work you have to do, some of this has to do with making best use of your time. However, some of it has to do with managing the amount of information that you will collect, process and use within the evidence-based practice healthcare dissertation/final project or evidence-informed decision-making assignment. Managing files is one area that needs thought. There is also the area of managing your references so that you do not lose material and its original source. You also need to manage references either manually or through specially designed software programs (see Chapter 8) that will keep the details of material you have collected and allow you to reference it in the reference system you are required to use (usually Harvard).

Organising things in terms of what goes where

Try to let your computer to do as much work for you as possible in terms of accessing material, a source for reading on screen and writing directly on screen. Crucially, clearly label files and folders with names that accurately reflect the content. You will have successfully completed academic work in the past. Writing an evidence-based practice healthcare dissertation/final project or evidence-informed decision-making assignment is the same kind of work but at a different level.

Consolidating your ideas and activities by talking to others about it

Some university departments use action learning sets to encourage students to problem solve. It is through meeting and sharing information with others that facilitates the discussion of progress and problem-solving activities.

You need to decide where your strengths are at the moment and then decide which areas you need to work on and how you can improve. Certainly talking it over with a friend can help. You can also gain support from a supervisor, although they will expect you to take a certain amount of responsibility yourself for things. The remaining chapters of this book will help you navigate your way through this journey!

Reference

Rees, C. (2010) Searching and retrieving evidence to underpin nursing practice. In: K. Holland and C. Rees, *Nursing: Evidence-Based Practice Skills*, pp. 143–166. Oxford University Press, Oxford.

For further resources for this chapter visit the companion website at
  www.wiley.com/go/glasper/nursingdissertation2e

Chapter 11

Chapter 12 **Getting the most from your personal tutor**

Ellen Kitson-Reynolds
University of Southampton, UK

Scenario

Charlotte is about to embark on her final-year project and has been allocated a personal tutor. She is aware that this project is a significant piece of work that may or may not follow a traditional dissertation format. She is quite anxious as to what this will look like in reality. Charlotte is keen to get the most out of her personal tutor and with her learning difference she is wondering what to expect and is a little overawed at the workload. Generally, though, she is positive about the chance to work on a one-to-one basis with a knowledgeable member of academic staff and to achieve a successful outcome.

Before approaching your academic support

As soon as your module or assignment is introduced to you, start to think about suitable topic areas. You will need to identify something relevant to your area of clinical practice and something that excites you, as you will be 'living' with it for several weeks and possibly months. Talk to your peers and people you work alongside in clinical practice to really get an understanding of differing perspectives and realities as there may be concepts you have not considered at all. Talking about the project highlights the potential for it being an appropriate topic area and helps you to consider where the gaps in the knowledge and related practices are. This may help you to refine your thinking and guide a plan later with your personal tutor. You also gain confidence about your level of understanding and ability to undertake the project

This chapter is based on an earlier chapter by Judith Lathlean.

How to Write Your Nursing Dissertation, Second Edition.
Edited by Alan Glasper and Diane Carpenter.
© 2021 John Wiley & Sons Ltd. Published 2021 by John Wiley & Sons Ltd.
Companion website: www.wiley.com/go/glasper/nursingdissertation2e

overall as well as talking about your findings within a multiprofessional clinical and academic environment.

Start to read around the subject area starting broadly and refining as your ideas surface. It is acknowledged that 'Research is spending 6 hours reading 35 papers, so you can write one sentence containing 2 references' (Bryan Gaensler @scibry, 2019). Consider how best to organise your reading and your records of the references/papers you find. It is not uncommon to lose a vital reference or forget where you read something of value and then cannot include it in your overall project.

Have a really good understanding about the project and what the workload entails. Read the briefing fully and ensure to note and identify aspects that you may not fully understand. It is much better to ask upfront than assume what is required. Projects take many forms currently; you may be asked to produce a paper for publication alongside a portfolio of evidence, carry out a small research project, clinical audit, service evaluation, or quality improvement project, design a research protocol or undertake a traditional evidence-based project. Whatever it is, be clear that you understand what is required.

You may be undertaking this project as a stand-alone module or as part of an overall programme of education. You may have had a significant length of time away from your studies and returning to study may be challenging for you. Think about what support you need and what you can do for your own independent learning and where you need to seek support and guidance for the rest. Equally, you may also find this a helpful task to assist your planning regardless of perceived ability.

Activity 12.1
- Reflect on what learning style you have and how you work best.
- Consider if you work best under pressure or like to plan and start work early.
- Consider how this may impact on others around you.
- How do you experience working in group seminars compared to self-directed/independent working?
- Access your local library to identify study support activities and resources that may be of benefit to you.

Chapter 12

How to get started

It is best to start on a good footing with your personal tutor. Usually a personal tutor is allocated to you but sometimes you may have met a lecturer during your programme who seems very interested in your topic idea. If this is the case it is worth asking if they might be able to supervise you, especially if you feel you are on the same wavelength. Otherwise personal tutors are allocated according to their knowledge of the subject. Supervision may occur face to face, at a distance using multimedia, email or telephone, or via group supervision. Consider how you communicate effectively and what format would be most appropriate to your understanding and development.

You should take the initiative to contact them once you have their details. Do this early – the sooner you can get started, the more successful you are likely to be. This shows your personal tutor that you are eager to start on your project and keen to get their support. It is also the beginning of a successful relationship and one that will help you to produce the best possible dissertation. Your first meeting may be about how to set up future meetings and if, like Charlotte, you have specific learning requirements (e.g. dyslexia and/or autism), it may be helpful to familiarise yourself with names, places and routines. Be transparent about any learning differences you may have as your personal tutor will be able to work to your strengths.

Agreeing a working pattern

At the outset you may wish to draw up a research contract with your personal tutor and agree a method of contact, including how often you will meet, what you will do when you meet, and so on. This will aid the amicable negotiation of mutual expectations at the formative stages of supervision and helps avoid problems later in the supervision process. Be organised and plan early.

As you progress through the year, reflect and set goals with your personal tutor for your supervision meetings. Remember that they will not contact you. It is your responsibility and, above all, bear in mind that the chances of gaining a good degree or module grade without regular supervision are greatly reduced. You will undoubtedly be wanting feedback on your writing style and critical thinking skills development, so remember that the personal tutor will need time to read and/or respond to any electronic form of communication. This may be a negotiated time period of three to five days rather than the night before, unless agreed beforehand.

Anticipating and preventing problems

So, what gets in the way of a successful project? It is important to be realistic about access to your personal tutor. They want you to be successful and work with you, but equally they have other students to look after, usually heavy teaching loads and, if they are active researchers themselves, large research projects to manage. Agree with them how often you will be in contact and put it in your diary. Before you meet, many students find it helpful to prepare a short 'agenda' and after the meeting write a brief note of what you have agreed with your personal tutor.

It is vital to maintain a professional attitude to your project, as this will show your personal tutor that you are taking it seriously in both academic and clinical settings. Indeed, the project and dissertation count towards your classification as well as being an excellent way of learning about the research basis of your chosen topic.

It is natural to be anxious about doing well in your project, and some students are nervous about revealing their concerns to their personal tutor. However, the personal tutor will be familiar with this and is there as much to help you with the emotional aspects of working on what may be, for you, an unfamiliar activity, as to provide subject knowledge.

Good planning is the essence

Developing a realistic plan, with manageable time scales, is the key to keeping a project on track. Your personal tutor will be able to help you with this, though the project and your ability to complete it is your responsibility. Many students find a Gantt chart helpful (see Chapter 1). This lists the main activities and the time periods involved (a typical chart is shown in Table 12.1).

The Gantt chart shows when you are seeing your personal tutor, when activities will take place, when chapters will be prepared and when the personal tutor can expect to get some written material sent to them in advance of your discussion. You may also find it useful to set up your electronic calendar to remind you of deadlines and to send calendar invites to your personal tutor for when they should expect pieces of work to review and any meetings due.

Preparation of the chart needs you to develop a logical structure for your work. It also implies that you have the knowledge required for the activities, such as the best databases for searching the literature, a critiquing tool such as CASP for handling the literature, and an understanding of the methodol-

Table 12.1   Sample Gantt chart.

Tasks	Month 1	Month 3/4/5	Month 6/7/8	Month 9/10	Month 12
See personal tutor	[?]	[?]	[?]	[?]	[?]
Literature searching	[?]	[?]	[?]	[?]	[?]
Critique papers	[?]	[?]	[?]	[?]	[?]
Write Chapter 1 and 2	[?]	[?]	[?]	[?]	[?]
See personal tutor	[?]	[?]	[?]	[?]	[?]
Write Chapter 3 and 4	[?]	[?]	[?]	[?]	[?]
See personal tutor/write Chapter 5	[?]	[?]	[?]	[?]	[?]
See personal tutor with draft dissertation	[?]	[?]	[?]	[?]	Finish

Chapter 12

ogy if, for example, you are primarily looking at randomised controlled trials. Again, your personal tutor may be able to help you, but also there are likely to be sessions in your course that address such aspects or books and articles that you can access to give extra guidance. Don't forget the library resources.

It is not the end of the world if you fall behind on your time plan, but if you find that you have, you will need to review time scales to get back on target for completion. Also factor in proofreading time at least a week before the submission is due.

Supervision at a distance

Although your supervision may be face to face, increasingly students need to make use of other resources too, such as email and other forms of digital communication including video calls. Access to technologies is changing at a fast pace and not all individuals have access to all types of modern communications. Communication between individuals and groups has been transformed since the inception of electronic means. However, email must be used wisely. If you have a draft chapter to present to your personal tutor for feedback, a good way of conveying it is by email. Nevertheless, do not expect your personal tutor to read it and give you feedback by return. A realistic turnaround time should be negotiated with your personal tutor at the outset and re-confirmed at various stages during the period of supervision. Many personal tutors are prepared to organise video or telephone sessions when meeting in person is not possible.

Additional support

The personal tutor is there to give you support in your project; however, it is expected that you will be able to make the most of this support yourself by

---

Activity 12.2

Imagine that you are undertaking your own project. Your nursing associate colleague in a neighbouring clinical area, Alisha, is undertaking a module on her programme and over coffee one day you find that her topic is almost identical to the one you did in the past and have subsequently built upon! You check it out with her and her main personal tutor and it is agreed that you will act as more than a peer – rather than a co-supervisor for her project.

So what can you expect from Alisha and she from you in this role? The answers may be found in this chapter and you can add to them (Box 12.1). Thinking about yourself as a peer support should give insight as to how you could relate to your own personal tutor.

> **Box 12.1 Helpful additional suggestions**
> - In agreeing to be a peer support, you have a responsibility towards Alisha. Equally this is her project and not yours!
> - If you agree a certain pattern of working with her, try to keep to it unless circumstances change for either of you. In turn you should also expect respect from her; for example, giving you ample warning of problems that are preventing her from progressing or her inability to attend a planned meeting.
> - Look for the positives, firstly in her work and then in how she can improve, rather than seeking to critique or criticise her ideas alone. She should expect from you 'balanced' feedback.
> - Although Alisha does not have a specific supervisor, she does have the opportunity to book one-to-one sessions with her module lead by appointment and this may be something to consider when planning peer support.
>
> Above all, enjoy working with her. The relationship is likely to have some reciprocity. Whilst you will know more than the supervisee, a peer support can learn something new from every person supervised.

being organised and taking responsibility for your own learning. Many resources are at your disposal, through a whole variety of means. Also, turn to your peers and colleagues; they, too, may have some useful hints, tips and advice.

Resources

Critical Appraisal Skills Programme (CASP), https://casp-uk.net/.

For further resources for this chapter visit the companion website at
www.wiley.com/go/glasper/nursingdissertation2e

Chapter 12

Section 4 **Preparing to use research evidence in your dissertation**

At this point Sam is looking for qualitative studies to use in his dissertation and Sue is looking for randomised controlled trials that will help her answer her dissertation question. One of Sue's friends wants to examine historical literature. Alisha thinks she will need both qualitative and quantitative studies to support her topic and Charlotte is searching for systematic reviews and meta-analyses as well as randomised controlled trials.

Chapter 13 Clinical standards, audit and inspection

Diane Carpenter[1] and Alan Glasper[2]
[1]*University of Plymouth, UK*
[2]*University of Southampton, UK*

Scenario

Charlotte and Alisha have been discussing how successful or unsuccessful colleagues have been at making changes in practice based on best evidence. Both are keen to see how policies, audit, governance and healthcare regulation fit into evidence-based practice. Charlotte's 7000-word final written report has to demonstrate her ability to develop a plan to improve an aspect of professional practice. This includes identifying and justifying a clinical issue, critically appraising clinical guideline recommendations that address this issue, and importantly designing a clinical audit which aims to improve practice. Alisha for her assignment specifically needs to demonstrate an understanding of the clinical audit process as a way of measuring current healthcare provision. Sam and Sue both have to consider data from national audits as part of their search of the grey literature.

It is important to stress that healthcare professionals need a good working knowledge of how healthcare is regulated and how it deals with quality assurance matters. Crucially, all healthcare practitioners should see governance activities as part of the toolkit of essential life skills they need for professional practice irrespective of their discipline. Additionally, it is important to have a good understanding of how to integrate the theory of governance with other subject areas and reflect on how this informs practice in the delivery of holistic care in a patient-led health service.

This chapter is based on an earlier chapter by Alan Glasper and Colin Rees.

How to Write Your Nursing Dissertation, Second Edition.
Edited by Alan Glasper and Diane Carpenter.
© 2021 John Wiley & Sons Ltd. Published 2021 by John Wiley & Sons Ltd.
Companion website: www.wiley.com/go/glasper/nursingdissertation2e

This chapter covers the following elements.

- Healthcare governance and factors that enhance or detract from effective governance.
- The role of external auditors such as the Care Quality Commission (CQC) in England and the National Institute for Health and Care Excellence (NICE).
- The role of healthcare professionals in designing and implementing audit tools to measure compliance with local and national benchmarked care standards.
- The role of regulatory healthcare bodies and how they ensure that healthcare professionals are fit for practice and purpose fit for public protection.
- How adverse incidents are managed in healthcare settings.

What is healthcare governance?

Clinical governance, as healthcare governance is commonly known in the UK, lies at the heart of most health services. Healthcare governance exists to develop a modern, patient-led health service that delivers high-quality and safe client patient care. The report of the Francis Inquiry (2013), which examined the causes of the failings in care at the Mid Staffordshire NHS Foundation Trust between 2005 and 2009, represented perhaps the most in-depth analysis of a modern health service and systems and made a number of key recommendations; subsequently, many national initiatives in governance emerged.

Scally and Donaldson (1998) describe the antecedents to clinical governance which were partly based on concerns about the quality of care being delivered to patients and their families. Politicians of all parties have been at pains to stress that the NHS takes quality issues seriously. Scally and Donaldson (1998) define clinical governance as:

A framework through which NHS organisations are accountable for continuously improving the quality of their services and safeguarding high standards of care by creating an environment in which excellence in clinical care will flourish.

Healthcare services should therefore be:

1. efficient
2. effective
3. economic.

Halligan and Donaldson (2001) point out that governance belongs to all who work in health services not just doctors and nurses. This means that all staff members need to feel valued and part of the bigger picture. Governance should not be a top-down heavy-handed approach by governments but a shared philosophy in which all professionals can contribute as they deliver the best standard of care they can, while continually seeking improvement. Clinical governance is used to ensure safe, high-quality care from all involved in the patient's journey and ensure that the client remains at the centre of the activities which support governance.

There are a number of components to clinical governance, including:

- patient, public and carer involvement;
- risk management (incident reporting, infection control, prevention and control of risk);
- staff management and performance (recruitment, workforce planning, appraisals);
- education, training and continuous professional development, professional re-validation, management development, confidentiality and data protection;
- clinical effectiveness (clinical audit management, planning and monitoring, learning through research and audit);
- information management (patient records, etc.);
- communication (with patients and the public, external partners, internal, board and organisation wide);
- leadership (throughout the organisation, including Board, Chair and non-executive directors, chief executive and executive directors, managers and clinicians);
- team working (within the service, senior managers, clinical and multidisciplinary teams, and across organisations).

At the heart of clinical governance lies a mission to ensure patient safety, provide the highest quality of care and promote lifelong learning among healthcare staff. Crucially, clinical governance belongs to everybody who works in a healthcare organisation.

It can be argued that the care patients and clients receive is only ever as good as the healthcare professional who delivers it. Healthcare staff are usually the first point of contact with patients and that is why communication theory features so strongly in healthcare curricula, where the recognition that simple non-verbal communication such as a smile can have major positive effects on worried patients or relatives. Clinical governance therefore encompasses everything concerned with quality care from the simple to the complex but at its heart lies a mission to deliver patient-focused care in which

Chapter 13

the culture of the healthcare setting is effective, efficient and, importantly, economic (sometimes called the three Es), although governance is not just about saving money!

In the world of healthcare, which is regularly scrutinised by the media and politicians alike, it is crucial that those who work in this highly visible environment have a full understanding of what governance is and, importantly, how to use it for better patient care.

What are the seven pillars of clinical governance? Are they still relevant in contemporary practice?

The Seven Pillars of Clinical Governance model first articulated by the NHS Clinical Governance Support Team in 1999 has been adopted by many clinical environments ever since to coordinate their governance activities. The pillars are still perceived to be relevant and the pinnacle of sound governance is the 'partnership' between the patient and the healthcare professional as they each strive to achieve optimum healthcare. The personal traits of the healthcare professional and how they act cements or demolishes the patient's perspectives of the care given, not only of the professional who has delivered the care but also the host organisation. If partnership in care is to be truly embraced by staff, the organisation as part of its governance activities must embrace notions of patient and public involvement with all aspects of healthcare planning and delivery.

The Seven Pillars
1. Clinical effectiveness
2. Risk management
3. Patient experience
4. Communication effectiveness
5. Resource effectiveness
6. Strategic effectiveness
7. Learning effectiveness

The pillars are supported by five foundation stones.

1. Systems awareness
2. Teamwork
3. Communication
4. Ownership
5. Leadership

These foundation principles underpin the whole edifice of governance and need to be regularly inspected to ensure that the pillars remain secure. Each of the pillars is dependent on the others and if one pillar does not deliver its commitment to the principles enshrined in governance then the whole structure collapses. Hence, healthcare governance activity cannot be cherry-picked. Investigations carried out by the Healthcare Commission (2005), now the CQC, and the government report of the Mid Staffordshire NHS Foundation Trust public inquiry (Francis, 2013) remind healthcare professionals of the consequences of what happens when governance pillars, such as communication, and foundation stones, such as are teamwork and leadership, come crashing down.

The role of the Care Quality Commission

The CQC was created in 2009 following the merger of three former regulatory organisations, namely the Health Care Commission better known by healthcare professionals as the Commission for Healthcare Audit and Inspection (CHAI), the Commission for Social Care Inspection and the Mental Health Act Commission. The primary function of the CQC is to regulate and inspect health and social care services in England. The CQC achieves this by conducting audit inspections through which they assess compliance with their standards.

In context to the evolution of CQC hospital inspections, the Francis Inquiry report was published on 6 February 2013 and examined the causes of the failings in care at Mid Staffordshire NHS Foundation Trust between 2005 and 2009 (https://www.gov.uk/government/publications/report-of-the-mid-staffordshire-nhs-foundation-trust-public-inquiry).

This public inquiry report was critical of role of the Healthcare Commission which was the NHS regulator in England until April 2009 and the Care Quality Commission which replaced it in the same month. Subsequent to the tragic events which occurred at the Mid Staffordshire NHS Foundation Trust, the CQC was motivated to introduce new and more rigorous hospital inspections designed to avert any future scandals. The post Francis Inquiry CQC inspections became not only more comprehensive but also temporally longer, typically lasting up to three days.

In contemporary healthcare the CQC's primary role is to ensure that hospitals in England provide service users with high-quality care, and to encourage them to take steps to continuously improve that care. To achieve this it is necessary for the CQC to solicit data from hospitals on a wide range of topics, but central to the process is risk-based regulation. As part of the regulatory process, risk can be explained as the risk of a hospital not achieving outcomes that the various healthcare policy standards, codes, regulations, etc. are designed to achieve and therefore the CQC uses a number of methods for gathering, analysing and understanding information,

Chapter 13

which helps them to identify the risks of poor care delivery in clinical environments.

In January 2010, the CQC introduced new essential standards and these are now the policy vehicle for the continued application of clinical governance to the health service in England. Clearly for clinical governance to work, practitioners need to ensure that the foundations are secure. Imagine the essential care standards as the expensive curtains at the window that is your healthcare environment. Clinical governance is the sound, clean and draught-proof window to which the curtains can be hung to their best advantage. Stained, faded and mildewed curtains soon expose the reality of the state of the building, in this case the institution.

The essential care standards have not been published to replace or succeed clinical governance. In fact, clinical governance has a vital role to play in ensuring that healthcare organisations can satisfy the demands of the healthcare watchdogs, such as the CQC in England, to monitor how institutions comply with these benchmarked standards and upon which future organisational performance measurement is estimated.

Background

The Health and Social Care Act 2008 received Royal assent on 22 July 2008 and the act thus established the CQC, which now is the principal regulator for health and adult social care in England, with stringent powers to ensure that safe and high-quality services are provided. Its primary mission is to facilitate improvements, champion the rights of the people who use services, acting promptly to address any poor or underperforming areas of practice and, crucially, gathering and sharing knowledge and expertise. This healthcare regulator ensures that the care people receive meets the essential standards of quality and safety. Methods to assess the veracity of the evidence include CQC inspection visits to individual healthcare establishments.

What are the essential standards of quality and safety?

The themes are grouped under six key areas, each of which has a number of specified outcomes (Table 13.1). The six key areas are subdivided into 28 discrete outcomes that the CQC expects patients and their families to experience if the individual English NHS Trust is to be compliant with its regulations. The CQC fully expects that all NHS trusts conform to these and that professionals understand its system for monitoring quality. Where there is evidence of adverse outcomes then the CQC will consider the action it needs to take to protect people's safety, dignity and rights.

Table 13.1   The essential standards of quality and safety.

Involvement and information (3 outcomes)

Outcome 1   Respecting and involving people who use services

Outcome 2   Consent to care and treatment

Outcome 3   Fees

Personalised care, treatment and support (3 outcomes)

Outcome 4   Care and welfare of people who use services

Outcome 5   Meeting nutritional needs

Outcome 6   Cooperating with other providers

Safeguarding and safety (5 outcomes)

Outcome 7   Safeguarding people who use services from abuse

Outcome 8   Cleanliness and infection control

Outcome 9   Management of medicines

Outcome 10   Safety and suitability of premises

Outcome 11   Safety, availability and suitability of equipment

Suitability of staffing (3 outcomes)

Outcome 12   Requirements relating to workers

Outcome 13   Staffing

Outcome 14   Supporting workers

Quality and management (7 outcomes)

Outcome 15   Statement of purpose (i.e. the primary aims of the Trust)

Outcome 16   Assessing and monitoring the quality of service provision

Outcome 17   Complaints

Outcome 18   Notification of death of a person who uses services

Outcome 19   Notification of death or unauthorised absence of a person who is detained or liable to be detained under the Mental Health Act 1983

Outcome 20   Notification of other incidents

Outcome 21   Records

Chapter 13

(*Continued*)

Table 13.1   (Continued)

Suitability of management (7 outcomes)	
Outcome 22	Requirements where the service provider is an individual or partnership (not applicable for NHS trusts)
Outcome 23	Requirement where the service provider is a body other than a partnership (i.e. requirements on NHS Trust chief executives)
Outcome 24	Requirements relating to registered managers
Outcome 25	Registered person: training
Outcome 26	Financial position
Outcome 27	Notifications: notice of absence (of service managers)
Outcome 28	Notifications: notice of changes (of service mangers)

How does the CQC in England operate?

The Commission uses the evidence related to compliance to the standard outcomes to determine:

- whether a healthcare provider continues to be suitable and is allowed to keep its registration with CQC;
- how individual providers comply with the essential standards of quality and safety;
- whether concerns about a healthcare provider should require it to make improvements or should prompt the Commission to use more formal powers, which include restricting, suspending or, in the most serious cases, removing a provider's registration.

Additionally, and importantly, the Commissioning for Quality and Innovation (CQUIN) payment framework (https://www.england.nhs.uk/nhs-standard-contract/cquin/cquin-20-21/) makes a proportion of providers' income conditional on quality and innovation and if healthcare providers achieve the outcomes there will be financial benefits.

The commission's assessment approach, together with its registration system, provide an immediate, credible picture of healthcare that promotes improvement and allows swift action to be taken where poor care exists. The CQC listens carefully to what people who use services report about their care and hold those in charge accountable when that care falls below optimum.

Most nurses working in hospitals will have either been directly or indirectly involved in a CQC inspection where a rating, ranging from outstanding, good, requires improvement to inadequate, is awarded for each of five key questions with equal weighting. The five key questions are as follows.

- Is the service safe?
- Is the service effective?
- Is the service caring?
- Is the service responsive?
- Is the service well-led?

Within the context of these key questions, inspection teams that include specialist advisors from the nursing profession endeavour to ascertain if the fundamental standards developed under the auspices of the Health and Social Care Act 2008 are met. These are:

- person-centred care (Regulation 9);
- dignity and respect (Regulation 10);
- premises and equipment (Regulation 15);
- receiving and acting on complaints (Regulation 16);
- good governance (Regulation 17);
- staffing (Regulation 18);
- fit and proper persons employed (Regulation 19).

The new CQC inspection regime was designed to avert any future scandal on the scale of the Mid Staffordshire NHS Trust tragedy. The new inspection process was introduced in 2014 and the CQC have seen many NHS Trusts make significant improvements in quality. The CQC believes that strong leadership and a positive open culture have been important drivers of change in these hospitals.

Nurses play not only a significant part in the hospital inspection processes but also a major role within their own hospitals in embracing the aspirations of the CQC and also the fundamental standards of care. As with the Nursing and Midwifery Council (NMC) code, nurses should intuitively reflect the CQC fundamental standards in their daily activities of providing excellence in care. Many nurses have been motivated to make innovations in care delivery and see CQC inspections as an excellent vehicle for cascading new and novel approaches to care to other organisations (Glasper, 2019).

What are the implications for nurses?

Nurses already play a major role in all aspects of quality patient care management and in reality the standards of the CQC actually complement those of other polices such as National Service Frameworks. There is no reason why audit tools which have previously been developed to measure compliance with

---

Scenario

Sue and Sam have been investigating the role of NICE in producing bench-marked standards.

---

policies such as the National Service Framework for Children, Young People and Maternity services (Coles *et al.*, 2007) should not be mapped against the CQC standards. Nurses have a good grasp and vision of what is required in audit processes and some have excellent user and carer initiatives already in place.

NICE quality standards

The first three NICE quality standards covering stroke care, dementia care and prevention of venous thromboembolism were presented to the Secretary of State on 30 June 2010. This work was being championed by the National Quality Board (NQB), which is a multistakeholder board established to promote quality across all aspects of the NHS and which is now part of NHS England. The variety of standards produced by NICE has the potential to subsequently become a crucial tool for supporting the commissioning and provision of high-quality services to patients. Furthermore, the NQB believes that these standards could become a central tenet of the whole quality improvement system for the NHS.

The role of the NICE quality standards

The National Institute for Health and Clinical Excellence was formed in 1999 and was originally tasked with setting standards for new health technologies (Pearson and Rawlins, 2005). Now known as the National Institute for Health and Care Excellence, NICE provides national guidance and advice to improve health and social care. For this purpose NICE used three stages – scoping, assessment and appraisal – to examine the evidence of the clinical effectiveness and cost-effectiveness of a particular technology in the NHS (Walker *et al.*, 2007). NICE has applied this expertise to the development of stringent standards. The quality standards developed by NICE have delineated an evidence-based and trustworthy vision of what high-quality care might resemble across the parameters of a pathway of care. These quality standards produced by NICE enable clinicians and clinical nursing teams to improve the quality of care being provided in the NHS. Over the years NICE aims to produce an inclusive across-fields-of-practice library of quality standards, covering all the main patient care pathways (http://www.nice.org.uk/aboutnice/qualitystandards/qualitystandards.jsp).

   The selection of topics, and the order in which the standards will be developed, is based on evidence in the following areas:

- quality of care (including experience), and potential to improve quality;
- cost to, and burden on, the NHS;
- prevalence, mortality and health burden on the population.

NICE and the NQB consider that these evidence-based and dependable descriptions of what high-quality care looks like across a pathway of care and in a format that can be understood by patients and the public can only be realised if the whole system, that is from individual clinical nursing teams right through to the national organisations responsible for the supervision, regulation and management of health and care services, declares support for their use. NICE quality standards are perceived to support clinical leaders by presenting them with the best available evidence in a clear and concise form, without taking away their freedom to make decisions that are in the best interest of their patients.

NICE quality standards have been designed to act as indicators across a whole pathway of care that is the healthcare journey that people with a specific condition go through in receiving care and treatment. To achieve this, a NICE quality standard may include quality statements relating to different types of care delivery, for example primary care from GPs and community nurses and acute care from doctors and nurses in hospitals.

How are NICE quality standards constructed?

To construct a standard, NICE establishes a multidisciplinary topic expert group on the clinical area being considered. Each group is then responsible for reviewing the available evidence-based academic literature from approved sources to initially identify 10–15 characteristics of high-quality care that define the quality standard for that topic. The topic expert group then deliberates and modifies the quality statements and eventually hones them down to a maximum of 10. Thus far, 187 (as of 2019) quality standards have been produced in conjunction with a range of supporting information to help nurses, among others in the NHS, to make best use of them as an instrument for delivering quality improvement.

A NICE quality standard is therefore a set of 5–10 specific, concise quality statements and associated measures that:

- act as markers of high-quality, clinically cost-effective patient care across a pathway or clinical area;
- are derived from the best available evidence from NICE guidance and other sources accredited by NHS Evidence;
- are produced collaboratively with the NHS and social care professionals, along with their partners and service users.

Chapter 13

NICE quality standards set out what clinicians, such as nurses, clinical teams, healthcare organisations and commissioners, should aspire towards. NICE quality standards describe what high quality should look like.

As an example, one of the standards published in 2010 gives detailed criteria statements pertinent to the care of patients suffering from dementia.

The NICE Quality Standard on dementia care

The NICE Quality Standard on dementia care consists of the following quality statements.

1. People with dementia receive care from staff appropriately trained in dementia care.
2. People with suspected dementia are referred to a memory assessment service specialising in the diagnosis and initial management of dementia.
3. People newly diagnosed with dementia and/or their carers receive written and verbal information about their condition, treatment and the support options in their local area.
4. People with dementia have an assessment and a continuous personalised care plan, agreed across health and social care, that identifies a named care coordinator and addresses their individual needs.
5. People with dementia, while they have capacity, have the opportunity to discuss and make decisions, together with their carer(s), about the use of advance statements, advance decisions to refuse treatment, Lasting Power of Attorney, Preferred Priorities of Care.
6. Carers of people with dementia are offered an assessment of emotional, psychological and social needs and, if accepted, receive tailored interventions identified by a care plan to address those needs.
7. People with dementia who develop non-cognitive symptoms that cause them significant distress or who develop behaviour that challenges are offered an assessment at an early opportunity to establish generating and aggravating factors. Interventions to improve such behaviour or distress should be recorded in their care plan.
8. People with suspected or known dementia using acute and general hospital inpatient services or emergency departments have access to a liaison service that specialises in the diagnosis and management of dementia and older people's mental health.
9. People in the later stages of dementia are assessed by primary care teams to identify and plan their palliative care needs.
10. Carers of people with dementia have access to a comprehensive range of respite/short-break services that meet the needs of both the carer and the person with dementia.

Importantly, in addition each of the quality statements for dementia care is backed up with the following.

- A *quality measure* consisting of both structure, in which evidence is sourced to demonstrate that institutions provide and maintain dementia training for staff, and process, in which the number of staff trained and who work with dementia patients is calculated.
- A *description* of what the quality statement means for each group involved, such as the nursing staff providing care or the individual patient who is a recipient of care.
- A *data source*, which also consists of structure (i.e. the audit tools to measure compliance) and process (i.e. how local data are collected).

How are NICE quality standards used in practice?
Both the NQB and NICE believe and are confident that the continuing production of the quality standards and their detailed criteria statements will:

- support clinical staff such as nurses in providing the best available evidence in a clear and concise format, without affecting their ability to make decisions in the best interests of their patients;
- empower patients, putting power and control into their hands around choice and clinical accountability;
- support local commissioners, in commissioning high-quality services, without losing their ability to commission innovatively, and in future.

NICE quality standards aim to enable:

- *healthcare professionals* such as nurses to make decisions about care based on the latest evidence and best practice;
- *patients* to understand what service they can expect from their nurses and other care providers;
- *healthcare organisations* to quickly and easily examine the clinical performance of their organisation and assess the standards of care provided;
- *commissioners* to be confident that the services they are providing are high quality and cost-effective.

Chapter 13

> **Scenario**
>
> Charlotte wants to design an audit tool to assess how her ward complies with one of the benchmarks detailed in a recent government healthcare policy.

Developing audit tools to measure compliance to policy standards

Implementing governance to ensure that policy standards are met usually involves undertaking an audit, which is a systematic and independent examination of how a healthcare organisation complies with local and/or national standards. Audit plays a key role in assessing how well an organisation is at meeting these set standards. Cooper and Benjamin (2004) believe that audit exists to improve the quality of patient care and clinical practice. Audit does this in a number of steps (Table 13.2).

Developing a local audit topic

Coles *et al.* (2007, 2010) reported measuring compliance with one of the standards of the children's national service framework and a range of other contemporary child health policy benchmarks in one English strategic health authority. They designed a tool that used a 5-point scale, with 1 indicating the lowest level of compliance and 5 the highest (Table 13.3). The audit results demonstrate that there were a number of areas that required further work before all the criteria of the standards were fully met within the specified period envisaged by the Department of Health.

Table 13.2   The audit cycle.

1	Selection of a topic (for example, pain management in patients)
2	Decide on criteria and standards (using, for example, the various policies related to pain management, see https://www.rcn.org.uk/library/subject-guides/pain)
3	Design and pilot the audit tool
4	Determine how the data or information will be collected (for example, how many patients' records will be surveyed?)
5	Collect the data following a strict time frame
6	Analyse the information and see if the results tally with the standards selected as the basis of the audit tool. Identify where compliance to the selected standards is suboptimal
7	Design and implement an action plan to address the areas of concern
8	Repeat the audit according to your action plan to monitor progress using the same audit tool

Scenario

Over coffee Alisha tells Charlotte about a journal paper she has read by Coles *et al.* (2010) who designed an audit tool to measure compliance with child health nursing policies.

Table 13.3 Audit tool segment example.

Benchmarks

1.1 Individualised Pain Assessment Tool for children in hospital

No pain assessment tool is available Score 1	Assessment tools are used and documented in less than 25% of records Score 2	Assessment tools are used and documented in 25–50% of records Score 3	Assessment tools are used and documented in 50–75% of records Score 4	Assessment tools are used and documented in 75–100% of records Score 5	If not applicable, please state why

Evidence (please indicate the presence or lack of evidence), for example:

- Paediatric pain assessment tool (state type). . . . .
- Neonatal pain assessment tool (state type). . . . .
- Completed pain assessment tools within patient records
- Pain audit results
- Other (please state)

Source: based on Coles *et al.* (2010).

Importantly, before setting out on the audit trail someone needs to become the audit lead. This person will liaise with the multidisciplinary team where necessary to ensure that the audit tool design is suitable for the topic under investigation. For maximum effect and to prevent non-cooperation, the auditing team should be peers rather than managers. This method will ensure maximum enthusiasm for the task ahead. The writers of policy and other similar documents usually couch their publications in such a way that the information embodied within can be easily converted into an audit tool.

It is important to remember that audit is designed to eventually produce an outcome for a patient or service-user group. Hence, in the design of the audit tool reference to benchmarking should be made. Many audit tools, such as the one cited above, use either a 5- or 10-point ordinal scale. The ordinal measurements only give information on order, as in, for example, bad to good, and do not in any sense describe the degree of difference between the items being measured, in this example how individual pain assessment tools are used for children in hospital settings. Although the scoring scale is ordinal, it still informs the practitioner undertaking the audit as to how an individual clinical area adheres to evidence-based practice guidelines and benchmarks contained in healthcare polices.

What exactly is benchmarking?

Benchmarking is simply comparing your practice against others offering similar services. For example, you might wish to compare your hand-washing audit results with those of another hospital. Thus benchmarking allows you as a practitioner or group of practitioners to compare yourself or your service with other similar organisations. The origin of benchmarking is lost in history but by the middle of the nineteenth century as the Industrial Revolution was at its peak in Western countries a standard measurement, for example screw length, had to be agreed and fixed to enable products or product components built in one part of the country to be interchangeable with each other. Hence, the mark on the craftsman's bench indicated the agreed size for the component in question, in this case a screw. Such practice allowed, for example, gun parts to be interchangeable, allowing repairs to be easily made on the battlefield.

Ellis (2000) has described how clinical benchmarking can help practitioners determine the evidence base on which the benchmarks for practice are agreed and, importantly, in accepting the status of a benchmark allow both measurement (in the form of scores often using a 10-cm visual analogue scale) and comparison and the sharing of best practice with other similar institutions of units. Benchmarked standards are now a key feature of many policy documents supported and triangulated with evidence from a number of sources. One key policy pertinent to all healthcare practitioners is Essence of Care (Department of Health, 2010). Essence of Care covers the 12 benchmarks that ensure best practice in healthcare and which are intended to stimulate healthcare practitioners to tackle their own patient/client issues of concern within their workplace with the specific intention of improving the services they provide.

Activity 13.1

Go to https://www.gov.uk/government/publications/essence-of-care-2010. Examine each of the 12 benchmarked Essence of Care standards. How would you compare your current practice with each one of these?

Healthcare regulators

Scenario

Sue has met a reviewer from the Nursing and Midwifery Council who was visiting her ward to discuss with mentors their role in supporting pre-registration nursing students.

The UK regulators of healthcare professionals
- General Chiropractic Council
- General Dental Council
- General Medical Council
- General Optical Council
- General Osteopathic Council
- Nursing and Midwifery Council
- Pharmaceutical Society of Northern Ireland
- Royal Pharmaceutical Society of Great Britain
- The Health Professions Council, which regulates no less than 15 health professions, including biomedical scientists, chiropodists/podiatrists, clinical scientists, dietitians, hearing aid dispensers, occupational therapists, operating department practitioners, orthoptists, paramedics, physiotherapists, practitioner psychologists, prosthetists/orthotists, radiographers, and speech and language therapists.

The role of healthcare regulators
All healthcare regulators are committed to protecting the public through professional standards. Regulators such as the NMC do this by:

Chapter 13

- setting standards;
- approving courses such as pre-registration nursing programmes;
- keeping and maintaining a register (for nurses, midwives and nursing associates);
- taking action against registrants when necessary.

All regulators, such as the General Medical Council, exercise this commitment to protect, promote and maintain the health and safety of the public by ensuring proper standards, in this example through the practice of medicine. When it fails, as in the case of Dr Harold Shipman, who was convicted of 15 murders but is thought to have killed 236 patients, the public has a right to be concerned (Horton, 2001). Similarly, an examination of the case of enrolled nurse Beverley Allitt reveals that the primary driver in solving the mystery of the unexplained deaths of children was harnessing the suspicions of other nurses and spurring them into actions which eventually exposed her crimes. MacDonald (1996) reveals that the nursing profession was appalled that while Allitt was employed on a six-month fixed-term contract on the children's ward at Grantham and Kesteven District General Hospital she murdered four children and injured nine others. Hence, healthcare regulators take great steps to ensure that there is no repetition of the Shipman or Allitt case.

The NMC was established under the Nursing and Midwifery Order (2001) and came into being on 1 April 2002 as the successor to the UKCC (United Kingdom Central Council) and the four National Boards. The NMC has a remit to deal with allegations made against nurses. Impairment of a nurse's fitness to practice could be due to:

- misconduct;
- lack of competence;
- conviction or caution for criminal offence;
- physical or mental health;
- fitness to practice deemed impaired by other regulatory body;
- incorrect or fraudulent entry in register.

The NMC and other regulatory bodies can exercise a number of sanctions against registrants who fail to comply or adhere to the professional code of conduct, in this example for nurses (Box 13.1). These sanctions include:

- interim suspension;
- interim conditions of practice;
- removal for at least five years;
- caution for one to five years;

Chapter 13

> **Box 13.1   The NMC code: standards of conduct, performance and ethics for nurses and midwives (updated 10 October 2018)**
>
> As a registered nurse or midwife the people in your care must be able to trust you with their health and well-being. To justify that trust, you must:
> - Make the care of people your first concern, treating them as individuals and respecting their dignity.
> - Work with others to protect and promote the health and well-being of those in your care, their families and carers, and the wider community.
> - Provide a high standard of practice and care at all times.
> - Be open and honest, act with integrity and uphold the reputation of your profession.
>
> These are the shared values of all healthcare professionals.

- suspension from register;
- conditions of practice.

How does the NMC function in contemporary healthcare?

The NMC regulates the nursing and midwifery and nursing associate professions in a number of discrete areas.

Public protection

Healthcare remains, and is likely to remain, a topic of heated debate within the public domain, with a growing emphasis on patient safety and the avoidance of adverse incidents and poor performing institutions, such as seen in the Mid-Staffordshire NHS Foundation Trust (Triggle, 2010). In order to fulfil its own commitment to public protection, which is at the very core of its activities, the NMC is factoring changes in demographics into its deliberations, to understand and predict the public's need for nurses and nursing care. This may therefore necessitate an increase in the number of registrants. Importantly, the population as a whole is ageing and is projected to have many more years of ill health than in earlier decades. This, in particular, will result in an increased demand for mental health and other related nursing services. Similarly, if rising trends in obesity, alcohol abuse and sexually transmitted diseases do not abate, the impact on community and public health nursing will need significant forward planning.

Nursing and midwifery

The regulation of the UK nursing profession is a highly complex operation. Of great concern to the NMC is the reality that a high proportion of registrants (i.e. one-third) is over 50 years of age. Additionally, although the

Chapter 13

majority of nurses work within the NHS, the growth in the number of those working in the voluntary and independent sector is predicted to rise. Importantly, being the dominant part of the workforce, nurses account for the largest part of NHS expenditure.

Regulatory sector

The NMC and its forerunners, the UKCC and the General Nursing Council (GNC), was hard fought for by the nurses of yesteryear and came into being in December 1919 as a result of the Nurses Registration Act. Although New Zealand was the first country to regulate nurses under the Nurses Registration Act of 1901, the NMC is now widely regarded as being one of the world's strongest nursing regulators.

The NMC is aware that it cannot remain in nursing and midwifery isolation comprising the UK alone, as the impact of leaving the European Union will have profound influences on the free movement of workers, including nurses.

Education and training

The educational remit of the NMC is highly complex and requires significant planning. Throughout the UK, higher education institutions provide education for nurses, midwives and nursing associates. Unlike other European countries, which mainly offer one level of nursing, the NMC, in addition to regulating the training of nursing associates and nurses from four fields of practice, also currently approves many specialist practitioner programmes, teaching programmes and prescribing programmes. Importantly, the NMC approves the training programmes for nurses, midwives and nursing associates, by far the biggest healthcare student groups in the NHS.

Policy initiatives

Changes to NHS policy can have a major impact on the nursing profession, and importantly for the NMC is the reality that each of the four countries of the UK produces individual and separate health policies and changes to the overall structure of the NHS. Structurally, for example, the health service in England led by an internal market model differs in context to that of, for example, integrated health and social care in Northern Ireland.

In England specifically, the NHS will become more patient led and the healthcare regulator, the CQC, will monitor this.

NMC performance

The NMC, like other healthcare regulators, is itself independently audited. Importantly, in 2010 the Council for Healthcare Regulatory Excellence (CHRE)(https://www.gov.uk/government/publications/council-for-healthcare-regulatory-excellence-annual-report-and-accounts-2010-to-2011-vol2) expressed concerns that the NMC had not always acted in ways that have protected the public or that would fully maintain public confidence in the professions which it regulates. The NMC responded positively to these criticisms in reviewing its own governance systems and in embracing new technology to improve operational performance.

The NMC is one of the most respected healthcare regulators in the world. In one form or another it has been serving the public and the profession for over 90 years. The NMC endeavours to consider all those elements that might positively or negatively impact on its primary mission, which is to protect the public by ensuring that nurses and midwives provide the highest standards of care to their patients and clients.

Responding to an adverse incident

Reason (1990) indicated that 10% of patients in hospital suffer an adverse incident during their period of care. The elderly, people with mental health problems or learning difficulties, and children are especially vulnerable and healthcare professionals working in these environments must consider the context in which they work and deliver care. The biggest proportion of incidents in acute care settings tends to be patient accidents (e.g. falls, especially in the elderly), incidents arising from treatments and procedures, drug errors, and case note or other documentation incidents. Given the high rate of procedures leading to an adverse incident, healthcare professionals must adhere to local policies and guidelines, which are formulated to reduce the chance of an adverse incident. Clinical protocols must be established on best evidence and, importantly, be updated regularly. Crucially, the staff which provide care must be educated to do so and their competency assessed through annual monitoring coordinated through personal development plans. An adverse incident can be defined as any healthcare occurrence which has led to unintended or unexplained harm to a patient. A near miss is defined as an occurrence which may have led to a patient being harmed, but either the mistake was aborted before harm occurred or no harm actually resulted by chance alone.

Harm may befall a patient in a healthcare setting because of a variety of care deficiencies, such as (Mathews, 2007):

- medication delivery;
- mismatching patients and their treatment;
- equipment error;
- working beyond competency;
- failure or delay to make an accurate diagnosis;

Chapter 13

- suboptimal handover;
- suboptimal continuity of care;
- failure to ensure follow-up of investigations;
- lack of awareness of local procedures and policies.

Practices to minimise adverse incidents

- Develop a healthcare governance forum and morbidity and mortality meetings where risk issues are discussed weekly or monthly. Mortality and morbidity meetings were developed in the NHS to review deaths and serious incidents and to provide hospital boards with the assurance that patients were not dying or suffering as a consequence of unsafe clinical practices.
- Establish a local lead for risk management activities.
- Regular review of adverse event reporting.
- Full investigation (root cause analysis) of all 'red' National Patient Safety Agency (NPSA) graded incidents.
- Evidence of lessons learnt/practice change, for example nasogastric tube checking, cannula dressings.
- Link to audit programme.

Scenario

Sam has been advised by his supervisor to regularly check the National Patient Safety Agency website for information on patient safety alerts (http://www. npsa.nhs.uk/).

References

Care Quality Commission (2010) *Criteria for assessing NHS Trusts in 2010. The implications for nurses.* The Care Quality Commission.

Coles, L., Glasper, E.A., Fitzgerald, C. *et al.* (2007) Measuring compliance to the NSF for children and young people in one English strategic health authority. *Journal of Children's and Young People's Nursing,* **1** (1), 7–15.

Coles, L., Glasper, A., Battrick, C. and Brown, S. (2010) Assessing NHS trusts' compliance with child health policy standards. *British Journal of Nursing,* **19** (19), 1218–1225.

Cooper, J. and Benjamin, M. (2004) Clinical audit in practice. *Nursing Standard,* **18** (28), 47–53.

Department of Health (2010) *Essence of Care: Benchmarks for the Fundamental Aspects of Care.* The Stationery Office, London. Available at https://www.gov.uk/government/publications/essence-of-care-2010

Chapter 13

Ellis, J. (2000) Sharing the evidence: clinical practice benchmarking to improve continuously the quality of care. *Journal of Advanced Nursing*, **32** (1), 215–225.

Francis, R. (2013) *Report of the Mid Staffordshire NHS Foundation Trust Public Inquiry.* The Stationery Office, London. Available at https://www.gov.uk/government/publications/report-of-the-mid-staffordshire-nhs-foundation-trust-public-inquiry

Glasper, A. (2019) Have CQC hospital inspections resulted in better quality care? *British Journal of Nursing*, **28** (10), 654–655.

Halligan, A. and Donaldson, L. (2001) Implementing clinical governance: turning vision into reality. *British Medical Journal*, **322**, 1413–1417.

Healthcare Commission (2005) *Patient Survey Report 2004: Young Patients.* Healthcare Commission, London. Available at http://www.nhssurveys.org/Filestore/CQC/YP_KF_2004.pdf

Horton, R. (2001) The real lessons from Harold Frederick Shipman. *Lancet*, **357** (9250), 82–83.

MacDonald, A. (1996) Responding to the results of the Beverly Allitt inquiry. *Nursing Times*, **92** (2), 23–25.

Mathews, P. (2007) Adverse incident reporting. In: E.A. Glasper, G. McEwing and J. Richardson (eds) *Oxford Handbook of Children's and Young People's Nursing*, pp. 896–897. Oxford University Press, Oxford.

Nursing and Midwifery Council (2020) *The Code: Professional Standards of Practice and Behaviour for Nurses, Midwives and Nursing Associates.* NMC, London. Available at https://www.nmc.org.uk/globalassets/sitedocuments/nmc-publications/nmc-code.pdf (accessed 27 August 2020).

Pearson, S.D. and Rawlins, M.D. (2005) Quality, innovation, and value for money. *Journal of the American Medical Association*, **294**, 2618–2622.

Reason, J. (1990) *Human Error.* Cambridge University Press, Cambridge.

Scally, G. and Donaldson, L. (1998) Clinical governance and the driver for quality improvement in the new NHS. *British Medical Journal*, **317**, 61–65.

Triggle, N. (2010) Public inquiry into scandal-hit Stafford Hospital. BBC News Online (9 June 2010). http://news.bbc.co.uk/2/hi/health/10274537.stm (accessed 30 May 2012).

Walker, S., Palmer, S. and Sculpher, M. (2007) The role of NICE technology appraisal in NHS rationing. *British Medical Bulletin*, **81–82** (1), 51–64.

For further resources for this chapter visit the companion website at
www.wiley.com/go/glasper/nursingdissertation2e

Chapter 13

Chapter 14 **Understanding quantitative research**

Diane Carpenter[1] and Alan Glasper[2]
[1]*University of Plymouth, UK*
[2]*University of Southampton, UK*

It is not easy to write an evidence-based practice healthcare dissertation/final project or evidence-informed decision-making assignment and get good marks without having an understanding of research. This is because research is the major form of convincing evidence you will need to examine and include in your work. However, research can be divided into many different forms; the two major divisions are between quantitative and qualitative research approaches. Your skill in examining an article in a journal will depend on your knowledge of the basic principles of each type. This is because there are major differences in how each type is carried out and how they should be evaluated. Although a subsequent chapter looks at critiquing research, this chapter provides important preliminary information on the way in which quantitative research approaches are conducted. This knowledge will then allow you to evaluate how well studies have followed the principles of this approach.

The primary aim of this chapter is to outline the features of a quantitative research approach and some of the characteristics that make it popular within evidence-based practice.

Is it a quantitative study?

The differences between quantitative and qualitative studies are so different that they are often referred to as two different paradigms, where 'paradigm' means 'world view' (Tappen, 2011). This means the thinking that goes with

This chapter is based on an earlier chapter by Alan Glasper and Colin Rees.

How to Write Your Nursing Dissertation, Second Edition.
Edited by Alan Glasper and Diane Carpenter.
© 2021 John Wiley & Sons Ltd. Published 2021 by John Wiley & Sons Ltd.
Companion website: www.wiley.com/go/glasper/nursingdissertation2e

each type of research approach differs to the extent that they are almost opposites, or at least the sets of ideas about them are quite some way apart. So, for instance, one of the beliefs of the quantitative paradigm is that research is the search for generalisable statements about the constant relationships that exist between variables. Data are seen as objective measurements that can be verified by those with the skills to carry out the measurements. Reality is seen as somehow 'out there' and available to researchers through measurement. The qualitative paradigm is different in the way that it feels that 'reality' is inside each of us and we need to construct it through the eyes of those in the setting. In this way there is a different perception of research as an activity and the actions of the researcher within it.

One of the first questions to answer when you locate an article is whether it is a research study. If it is research, it will involve the collection of data from people or things in a systematic way and will include clear sections on how the information was collected. Data are simply *information* but usually made up of *facts* or *numbers*, which are collected by researchers who use them to help decision making. These articles will contain a results section that will often include tables or figures, such as bar charts or pie charts, that summarise information collected by the authors and which form the answer to their question or study aim. It will not be a review of the literature, which is information collected by

---

Scenario

At the start of their evidence-based practice healthcare dissertation/final project or evidence-informed decision-making assignment the four students compared their knowledge on research methods. They all knew that much of the evidence they would spend time reading as part of their literature review would demand a lot of careful consideration where they would have to draw on their research knowledge. Sue's topic of larvae therapy for wound healing in older women with varicose leg ulcers is likely to involve a number of randomised controlled trials (RCTs). She is not looking forward to this because, firstly, she sometimes gets confused between the two terms 'quantitative' and 'qualitative', and, secondly, because RCTs require knowledge of statistical terms and principles. Charlotte also finds 'quantitative' and 'qualitative' difficult due to her dyslexia – the words look very similar, so she does not always notice the difference. Sam's focus is on the lived experience of families with a child with a chronic illness, and his dissertation will mainly draw on qualitative studies (covered in Chapter 15) but may still contain some quantitative studies to provide some background and clinical detail. All the students are looking for some pointers to help them understand how these two research approaches differ and what they may need to take into account when evaluating studies from each area.

other people. It will not be a summary of the research produced by people who have read the original research and it will not be audit, which relates to findings in one particular clinical setting on the level of service compared to a standard (Gerrish and Lacey, 2010). It will have clear headings, such as aim, method, results, discussion and conclusion, but these will relate to an activity involving the collection of information using a specific data-gathering tool.

One of the easiest ways of establishing if it is a quantitative study is to confirm whether it contains tables and figures produced from the results. Usually, you will find this a reasonably successful method of identifying research type. This is based on the definition of quantitative research provided by Burns and Grove (2009:22) who defined it as:

> *a formal, objective, systematic process in which numerical data are used to obtain information about the world. This research method is used to describe variables, examine relationships among variables and determine cause-and-effect interactions between variables.*

This comprehensive definition highlights that the goal of the quantitative researcher is to turn the data gathered, if it is not already in that form, into a number. So height, temperature, number of children, and so on are already in the form of numbers but degree of pain, consciousness or anxiety have to be turned into a number using some kind of scale. This is one of the essential principles of quantitative research.

Why quantitative?

The reason for choosing a quantitative approach is really about the nature of the question the research wants to answer. Topping (2010) agrees, saying the researcher will chose the approach most appropriate for the problem under investigation. If the question requires something to be measured or involves the search for possible relationships between measurable variables, then they will choose a quantitative approach. One of the main purposes of evidence-based practice is to provide the healthcare clinician with the evidence for best practice when there are options available. 'Best practice' is usually seen as an intervention that has the greatest success in improving a measurable clinical outcome, such as a lower level of pain, fewer incidents of readmission or a higher level of physical functioning. A measuring research approach, as provided by quantitative research, is therefore the obvious choice.

Types of quantitative studies

A quantitative approach is a broad term used to describe a number of research designs that produce numerical results. These include:

- surveys, which can be descriptive or correlational;
- experimental approaches, such as RCTs;
- quasi-experimental approaches, which are similar to RCTs but lack important elements.

The following sections outline some key characteristics of each of these approaches.

Surveys

Descriptive surveys involve a large sample of people, things or events. The purpose of this type of survey is to produce a picture or 'snapshot' in numbers so that the investigators have some idea of the quantity or size of something, such as the number of people with asthma in a population or the views of patients on different types of treatment options. The aim is to be more precise in the understanding of quantity in regard to events, behaviour and attitudes of a defined group (McKenna *et al.*, 2010). The results are likely to just be an indicator rather than an exact answer, as surveys rarely include the whole population but rather a sample of them.

Surveys can look for patterns of relationships amongst the characteristics examined by taking a correlation approach. Polit and Beck (2008:272) define correlation as 'a tendency for variation in one variable to be related to variation in another'. For example, is there a pattern that links the social class of people and the extent to which they are following recommended health practices, such as a set level of fresh fruit and vegetables per day, or a pattern between age and type of anaesthesia people would prefer for a certain operation? The purpose of this type of research is more sophisticated and complex than a simple broad descriptive approach, as it allows researchers to predict the number of people who may be more likely to want certain things or be more likely to behave in a certain way. However, the results are again likely to be an indicator and not an exact prediction, as such a pattern may not relate to all people all of the time but will give an idea of a general trend that will be better than no information.

Experimental

Each type of study becomes progressively more sophisticated and complex in its design. One of the most sophisticated types of study is the RCT, which comes under the heading of experimental approaches. The emphasis here is often on comparing alternative interventions to see which has the better outcome on a patient's health or recovery.

The experimental process involves a group of people (although it can be objects or events) being randomly allocated to either an experimental or control group. The experimental group receives the variable that the researcher wants to test and the control group commonly has either an alternative

intervention (a placebo, i.e. a non-active or 'sham' intervention or procedure), or no intervention. These all allow a comparison between the group
with the experimental intervention and what would have happened either
without that intervention or in comparison with an alternative.

The important aspect of an experiment is the large degree of control the
researcher has in introducing the key *independent variable* and ensuring that,
as far as possible, other variables that make a difference to the outcome or
dependent variable are either not present or are present in reasonably equal
amounts in both groups through the process of randomisation. For those in
an experimental study there should be an equal chance of ending up in either
the control or experimental study. Random number generators on computers
or good-quality electronic calculators are used to allocate subjects in RCTs.

Quasi-experimental

In some cases where randomising people between two treatment methods is
very difficult or raises ethical issues, a less precise form of experiment called
a quasi-experimental study is used. Here 'quasi' means 'almost' and looks like
an RCT with an experimental and control group but does not have people
randomly allocated to the two groups; instead it uses groups that already
exist, such as people on two different clinical settings who are already part of
those settings. So it is almost, but not quite, a randomised control group.

Whereas the analysis of the results using statistical techniques can indicate
a cause-and-effect relationship between the variables in an experimental
study, in quasi-experimental studies these techniques can only suggest a correlation or pattern between the variables. In this situation the influences of
other variables, including the composition of the group, cannot be ruled out.
This possibility is reduced through the process of randomisation in a 'true'
experimental design involving randomisation. In a quasi-experimental
design, individuals clearly do not have a fifty-fifty chance of being in the
experimental group as they are already in a group before the study begins.

In all quantitative research approaches the emphasis is on accuracy of the
measurements used. The tool used to measure the outcomes must be *reliable*
(i.e. it is consistent and produces stable results whoever is measuring) and
repeat measures would produce the same result if repeated immediately.
Reliability is an important concept in research and is demonstrated when the
researcher uses a tool used in a previous study that is known to measure
accurately, for example the Glasgow Coma Scale or HAD depression scale, or,
where no existing tool is available and the researcher designs one that is fit
for purpose, a pilot study is used to test its accuracy or reliability.

Once measurement has taken place, the results have to be processed
statistically to see if any relationships exist between the variables using the

numbers as a way of indicating this. Statistical tests will indicate the likely existence of a correlation or pattern between variables in a study. Other tests, called *tests of significance*, will establish if it is likely that a cause-and-effect relationship exists between the variables. A study that can indicate this kind of relationship is the most prized type of research in quantitative research and is often referred to as the *gold standard*, as so much care or control over the process is taken to make the study as accurate as possible. This then permits the results of a study to be generalised, where the results can confidently be applied to other similar situations.

The ability of RCTs to indicate generalisable cause-and-effect relationships explains their position towards the top of the hierarchy of evidence, which is a way of indicating levels of preference for the type of studies chosen to answer an evidence-based practice question. At the top of the hierarchy of evidence are systematic reviews of RCTs, because of the care taken to produce these reviews by only including the most accurate and rigorous research available, which tends to be RCTs. Naturally for dissertation work it is these kinds of studies that would be the first choice, as they allow a student to argue for the use of a particular nursing intervention.

It is important to remember that if a systematic review on a certain subject has recently been published, it may prohibit the student from actually continuing with the evidence-based practice question which they have posed. This is because systematic reviews reassemble the parameters of some dissertation guidelines (but usually much more deeply) and as the whole purpose of completing a dissertation is to learn the skills of searching and critiquing literature, the existence of a recently published systematic review which does just that would undermine this.

Key elements in a quantitative study

When reading a quantitative study there are a number of elements you need to consider that will indicate the quality of the study and its relevance to your dissertation. These are covered further in Chapter 15 on critically appraising evidence, so only preliminary points are included here.

Having established that it is a research study, and confirmed it is a quantitative design by the presence of numbers either in tables or in the results section, look for the elements identified in Table 14.1. The table uses some of the familiar research terms you will meet in research studies and these are the words that will indicate your understanding of research in your dissertation. Using them will help you achieve better marks.

Table 14.1 provides you with a guide to the structure of most articles and the elements that you need to locate and consider. They will help you build

Table 14.1 Key elements in a quantitative study.

Element	Section where found	Why important	Look for
Variable(s)	Title, abstract, introduction, results	Helps confirm it matches key variable(s) in your work	How variables are defined and measured (concept and operational definitions). Compare these to other studies
Aim	Abstract, just before or after heading 'Methods' or similar term	This identifies what the researcher is trying to achieve through collecting data	Will this help the purpose of your dissertation? Compare this to other studies to check if they look at similar questions
Type of study or research design	Title, abstract, methods	Within quantitative and qualitative designs, each type has its own 'brand' appearance and follows clear principles	Although some studies will say 'qualitative' few say 'quantitative', but will indicate if it is a survey, experimental, randomised controlled trial (RCT), quasi-experimental, correlation or correlational design. Does it match the aim?
Research method/tool of data collection	Abstract, methods	Shows how data were collected	Is it appropriate for aim, approach, and sample? How accurate or reliable is it? Was accuracy checked by using a previously used tool or through a pilot?
Sample	Abstract, methods	Problems of bias or lack of convincing evidence can be related to the size of sample and way they were chosen	Clear inclusion and exclusion criteria, statement of sampling method. Size of sample should take into account variations in population and allow convincing results. Is sample relevant to aim and your dissertation? Is anyone not covered in criteria that might affect relevance? Is size of sample comparable to other studies and seems sufficient? Is method of choosing sample clearly described? Is size of those 'lost' to the study or not responding to the study a problem?

Ethical approval	Methods	Ethical issues raised by the process of recruiting people, or what is done to them. Check for mention of an ethics committee or IRB if any concerns
Results	Abstract, results	Are the results convincing or are there any limitations or uncertainties? Does this help answer your dissertation aim?
Tables, figures, text figures	Results	Will indicate part of answer to aim and statistical test values will indicate any relationships. Story suggested by figures. Good statistical values, e.g. $P < 0.05$, or better, e.g. $P < 0.01$
Main findings	In any tables or figures and text of the results section	Answers the aim of the study. Do the results build up to a clear answer to the aim which provides you with evidence for your dissertation
Conclusion	Abstract, end of discussion under heading 'Conclusion'	Will answer aim; anything that includes 'should' is a recommendation not a conclusion. Compare with other studies. Positive results to support your dissertation aim
Recommendations	Abstract and after conclusion	Will suggest 'best practice' and implications for practice. Statements containing 'should' as these indicate a recommendation. Compare these with other studies. Support your 'change' section and 'application to practice' in your dissertation

up a picture of the similarities and differences in studies you have found and enable you to start the critiquing process.

Strengths of quantitative studies

Quantitative studies are seen as the most desirable form of evidence for evidence-based practice. This is because of the many principles followed by quantitative researchers, such as the use of accurate measuring tools, which provides objective and visible outcomes similar to other scientific disciplines such as physics and chemistry. The method of collecting data in these studies is described in detail so that they can be repeated or reproduced to check for accuracy and rigour. In this way, high-quality 'rigorous' studies – ones that show the researcher's ability to produce accurate results – allow us to generalise the conclusion to other settings as care is taken in making the sample as close as possible to the larger group they represent.

Limitations

Despite the strengths noted previously, quantitative research also has limitations. For example, not everything that should be taken into account when deciding between alternative interventions is based on measurable outcomes. There are other considerations, such as the quality of care, or the wishes of the individual for the kind of intervention or, indeed, whether they will accept an intervention, that are just as important. In other words, quantitative results are only a part of the picture.

Some studies lack the rigour required to make the results strong enough to consider, often due to too small a sample or aspects of the study that have introduced bias into the results and conclusion.

Conclusion

Quantitative research is a major element in evidence-based practice because of its emphasis on accuracy and transparent methods of data collection. Knowing the structure and principles of the major forms of quantitative research will help you answer dissertation questions that relate to best practice. The gold standard for this kind of approach is the RCT, as this demonstrates the greatest degree of control by the researcher. It is also the method that indicates cause-and-effect relationships that allow clinical options to be chosen with reasonable confidence. Each study should be carefully examined to ensure that it conforms to the methodological principles of this kind of study. Although quantitative approaches have many advantages, there are still aspects that in healthcare need the balance provided by qualitative approaches. This research design forms the subject of Chapter 15.

References

Burns, N. and Grove, S. (2009) *The Practice of Nursing Research: Appraisal, Synthesis, and Generation of Evidence*, 6th edn. Saunders, St. Louis, MO.

Gerrish, K. and Lacey, A. (eds) (2010) *The Research Process in Nursing*, 6th edn. John Wiley & Sons, Chichester.

McKenna, H., Hasson, F. and Keeney, S. (2010) Surveys. In: K. Gerrish and A. Lacey (eds) *The Research Process in Nursing*, 6th edn, pp. 216–226. John Wiley & Sons, Chichester.

Polit, D. and Beck, C. (2008) *Nursing Research: Generating and Assessing Evidence for Nursing Practice*, 8th edn. Lippincott Williams & Wilkins, Philadelphia, PA.

Tappen, R. (2011) *Advanced Nursing Research: From Theory to Practice*. Jones and Bartlett Learning, Sudbury.

Topping, A. (2010) The quantitative–qualitative continuum. In: K. Gerrish and A. Lacey (eds) *The Research Process in Nursing*, 6th edn, pp. 129–141. John Wiley & Sons, Chichester.

For further resources for this chapter visit the companion website at
www.wiley.com/go/glasper/nursingdissertation2e

Chapter 15 **Understanding qualitative research**

Diane Carpenter[1] and Alan Glasper[2]
[1]*University of Plymouth, UK*
[2]*University of Southampton, UK*

In this chapter we will examine the second major paradigm used in healthcare decision making, that of qualitative research. This is a different way of thinking about research and how a study is conducted compared to that of quantitative research. The choice of which method to use is dictated by the nature of the research question the investigator is trying to answer. It is important that each approach follows a systematic and clear method that is described for the reader to judge the quality of the study outcome.

Scenario

Sam is trying to develop a better understanding of qualitative research methods as his dissertation examines the lived experience of families with a child with a chronic illness. He has chosen this topic as he wants to explore some of the issues that such families face. He knows that the term 'lived experience' is related to a phenomenological qualitative approach to research, but the terminology itself is very scary. He is trying to sort out how qualitative research differs from quantitative and he has read some very dismissive comments about this type of research. He feels that until he has a better understanding it is difficult to carry on with examining qualitative research with confidence. Sue is interested in the lived experiences of people who are undergoing larvae therapy as treatment for varicose ulceration of the legs. Charlotte as part of her project has to design a clinical audit that aims to improve practice by

---

This chapter is based on an earlier chapter by Alan Glasper and Colin Rees.

How to Write Your Nursing Dissertation, Second Edition.
Edited by Alan Glasper and Diane Carpenter.
© 2021 John Wiley & Sons Ltd. Published 2021 by John Wiley & Sons Ltd.
Companion website: www.wiley.com/go/glasper/nursingdissertation2e

reflecting guideline recommendations. She is interested in pain assessment and is seeking to more fully understand the Faculty of Pain Medicine (2015) core standards for pain management services in the UK, which have been formulated by the Royal College of Anaesthetists. Alisha has to demonstrate through a 2000-word literature review her knowledge and understanding regarding the research process that underpins contemporary evidence-based practice. She is considering examining the research that has been undertaken into optimising the timely and appropriate discharge of frail elderly patients from hospital.

One of the problems with qualitative research is that, as the spelling suggests, it concentrates on 'quality' issues, when it is more accurate to say it looks at experiences, interpretations and understandings as defined by those involved in a study. Whereas quantitative research can look at inanimate objects such as types of thermometers, walking aids, mattresses or methods of teaching, qualitative research always involves human beings. Holloway and Wheeler (2010:3) define qualitative research simply as 'a form of social inquiry that focuses on the way people make sense of their experiences and the world in which they live'. This emphasises many of the aspects of qualitative research, such as concentrating on how people themselves define a situation. They are not asked to choose from a number of alternatives, as in a questionnaire constructed from how a researcher interprets the world and what may be important. Qualitative research attempts to see the world through the eyes and interpretations of those in a particular situation.

The data gathered in qualitative research are usually in the form of words and that is how they are presented in a section typically called 'findings' as opposed to 'results', although this convention can sometimes be broken, often in ignorance or because of the conventions of the journal in which the study appears. As qualitative research does not 'count' anything or use a measuring tool to statistically examine numeric relationships between variables, there are no tables of figures forming the results, apart from a description of the characteristics of the sample. The whole way of thinking about this type of research is therefore different. This has led some supporters of a quantitative approach to research methods to reject the value of qualitative research in sometimes quite dismissive or 'name-calling' ways (Tappen, 2011:35). Again this is often more as a result of a lack of understanding of both the systematic way such research is undertaken and the value it can provide to healthcare decision making.

Why qualitative?

Qualitative approaches to both research and nursing have a clear compatibility. This is brought out by Holloway and Wheeler (2010:11) when they point out that it takes 'a person-centred and holistic perspective', which is the same as the approach of healthcare professionals such as nurses to individual care. This approach provides insight into the experiences of patients and clients of health services so that practitioners who have not experienced particular situations can begin to appreciate how it is for those concerned and provide a more sensitive and understanding form of care.

This approach does not replace but rather provides the balance or triangulation to a quantitative research approach. Although it is sometimes criticised for being very subjective and very descriptive, it is carried out in the same rigorous way as quantitative approaches, following clear principles of research with an emphasis on the accuracy of the findings.

Types of qualitative studies

As with quantitative approaches, there are a number of different designs grouped under the heading of qualitative research. Although there are many variations, there are three main types that predominate in nursing:

- phenomenology
- ethnography
- grounded theory.

There is also a fourth 'general' category that can be said to follow the general principles of qualitative approaches but does not follow any one approach in particular.

Phenomenology

This approach has developed from philosophy where there is an emphasis on an individual's lived experience of a situation. Often this kind of study will incorporate 'lived experience' into its title or aim; it is the approach that Sam is looking at in his dissertation and Alisha in her literature review that will consider how elderly people feel when their discharge back to the community is delayed. The method of data collection frequently used in this approach is in-depth interviews. They are not a question-and-answer format like a questionnaire but follow a very general opening such as 'Tell me what it is like to be the parent of a child with asthma', and then further questions will depend on what the respondent says. The follow-up questions will usually be requests for more details or illustrations of a point. There can be a loose structure of key topic areas to be covered in an interview but the aim is to produce spontaneous thoughts, interpretations or descriptions with the minimum of prompting from the interviewer. This conforms to the unstructured and flexible nature of qualitative methods (Tappen, 2011), where the intention is to capture rich detailed data in the respondent's own words. These lengthy verbal details produced in interviews are then analysed for common themes that emerge within them.

As with all these qualitative approaches, there are a number of variations within each one and you will find different models or guides being followed. Names such as Husserl and Heidegger, who developed the thinking on the philosophy of phenomenology, may appear, and Giorgi, Colaizzi or Van Manen may be cited in relation to the methodology, particularly in relation to the analysis of the data.

Ethnography

This type of study involves the observation of groups of individuals who share a common 'culture' in order to understand their pattern of behaviour. Often referred to as gathering data in 'the field', this type of research developed from anthropologists whose aim was to make sense of and describe the culture of remote tribes. In healthcare this has been used to look at the culture of different patient groups and even staff groups. Data are collected over periods of weeks, months or even years and consist of more than one form of data collection, such as observation, interviews and documentary methods. Researchers frequently keep a 'field diary' where their own thoughts, feelings and interpretations are captured and become part of the analysis and interpretation of the setting and its events.

The key to this kind of research is in the analysis, where themes emerge from the rich 'thick' descriptions (Holloway and Wheeler, 2010) using a structured form of analysis that is usually carefully described. In common with all forms of qualitative research this analytical approach takes an *inductive* approach, where the pieces of data are put together to form a view or interpretation of what it going on in a 'bottom-up' sequence.

Grounded theory

Whereas the last two types of research attempt to *describe* human situations and issues, the grounded theory approach, developed by two sociologists, Glaser and Strauss, attempts to *explain* or develop a theory to fit the situation. This theory is 'grounded' in the data that has been collected. Such studies sometimes express the theory in the form of a diagram that shows how all the ideas in the study fit together. In the same flexible, indicative process as previous approaches, it uses a mix of interviews, observation and documentary sources to construct its findings.

Key elements in a qualitative study

The differences between quantitative and qualitative studies can appear quite stark, as almost every aspect can look different. The two constants are the close attention to ethical rigour, where the same guidelines for the relationships between researcher and those involved in a study are protected, and on the outcome of the study matching the data collected as closely as possible. Both of these can be referred to as the rigour of the researcher in carrying out the study to the highest possible standards to ensure that quality of the results.

The key elements of a qualitative study revolve around the attempt to construct a view of the social world of the participants in a study from their own perspective and by concentrating on the richness and depth of information that is possible from the processes involved.

As shown in Table 15.1, which compares the two approaches, each aspect of the research process demonstrates differences. Firstly, the research question is broader and more general. Sample sizes are usually smaller as the emphasis is on the depth of data collected from each person. The sampling method does not try to match the sample to the population in the same way as quantitative research. The tool of data collection is far more flexible and does not attempt to be standardised, as it is not accurately measuring something but responding to capturing experiences or interpretations. This means the method of analysis in working with text or observations is very different, although frequently very systematic and follows the processes outlined by key writers of this type of research, such as Giorgi, Colaizzi or Van Manen. There is often the use of more than one tool of data collection to try to capture different aspects of the topic. This results in a certain amount of blending of findings in order to build up a clearer picture of the topic.

The interpretation of the data means that the thinking of the researcher follows a more inductive approach, building up to the suggestion of a bigger picture or theory rather than the deductive approach of quantitative research, which often attempts to apply a theory or bigger picture to the data to establish support for such a theory.

Strengths of qualitative studies

The major strength of qualitative studies is that they provide a rich and productive insight into human experiences in relation to health and illness. This produces a depth of understanding of human experiences (Houser, 2008).

Table 15.1 Comparison between key aspects of quantitative and qualitative research approaches.

Element	Quantitative	Qualitative
Aim	Specific and measurable	Broad question not answerable numerically
Purpose	Provide accurate answers to questions often involving the relationship between variables, either in a correlational or cause-and-effect relationship. Seeks to provide an 'answer' to a clear problem that can be generalised to other situations	Provide insights, experiences and interpretations. Seeks to provide variations in the way that people experience key health issues. Does not set out to generalise findings but increase understanding
Ethical considerations	Great emphasis placed on confidentiality, avoiding harm and gaining informed consent. If involving patients, particularly on health premises by health professional researchers, must get permission of an ethics committee	Same emphasis on doing no harm (including psychological or social), and gaining consent. However, as some studies do not involve patients on health premises, permission may not always be gathered from a health service ethics committee
Tool of data collection	Emphasis on accuracy and consistency of measurement to ensure standardisation of the tool	Often more than one tool used. There is flexibility in the use of the tool. In many respects the researcher almost becomes the tool of data collection through their dealings with people in the setting and recording what they see and hear
Viewpoint	The researcher's viewpoint drives the study through the power and control they have in the situation	The respondent's viewpoint is the major perspective used. This can be 'interpreted' through the researcher but they attempt to preserve the respondent's construction of how they see things
Method of analysis and data presentation	Objectively derived from statistical processes. Results are presented in the form of numbers	Researcher's interpretation of what they feel the data are saying. Systematic procedures followed in the analysis of the data. Findings are presented in the form of words, often under theme headings

(Continued)

Table 15.1   (Continued)

Element	Quantitative	Qualitative
Sample size and selection	Emphasis on large samples selected using processes that ensure they are closely representative of the total population they represent	Can be quite small but should have experienced the situation in which the researcher is interested. Selection procedures are less elaborate as generalisability is not an issue
Generalisability	Research processes should lead to high levels of generalisability	The aim is to heighten awareness of some situations but there is no primary emphasis on making them generalisable
Application to practice	High in relation to the question posed. Highly valued within evidence-based practice	High in relation to the question posed. Not highly valued in evidence-based practice but useful in issues of quality of care and ensuring a sensitive approach to individuals is achieved

This knowledge is quite different from that of quantitative studies as it is located more in the social world of health and illness rather than a medical model's focus on the body and the fight to regain health through interventions carried out by health professionals. The methods used by researchers are just as systematic as those of quantitative researchers, although very different in their characteristics, and the methodology sections of research articles should be just as transparent in revealing how the study was undertaken, especially the data analysis.

Limitations

Perhaps one of the greatest limitations of qualitative research is the mistrust amongst some health professionals that the conclusions of this type of research are not to be trusted because the interpretation of the findings are very much those of the researcher involved. Polit and Beck (2008:17) suggest that for some people the concern is whether two different qualitative researchers would reach the same conclusions from the same data. There is also the problem of whether findings can be generalised, as they are based on small samples.

The two major methods of interviews and observation popular in qualitative research also raise problems. Firstly, with interviews there is the difficulty of 'self-report' data, where there may be a difference between what people say they do and their beliefs and what they actually do and what their beliefs really are. In observational studies there is the problem of 'observer effect', where the presence of an observer may influence the behaviour of people being observed. An additional problem in observation is the inability of the researcher to 'see' everything and cover events or activities that are taking place simultaneously or in neighbouring locations. A certain amount of selection then is inevitable (Holloway and Wheeler, 2010).

Conclusion

Qualitative methods provide the balance to the more numeric and measurement orientated approach of quantitative research. The aim is to provide insights that allow nursing staff to provide a sensitive and insightful level of support. The holistic approach of the method is in keeping with that of nursing, which emphasises the total situation of the individual within their normal environment and not just the medical aspects of their life. This provides a depth of understanding that goes to the heart of the experience as described by those involved.

It is possible to have studies that combine quantitative and qualitative approaches, in mixed method studies. Here the aim is to provide balance and also to contribute to untangling frequently complex health situations (Simons and Lathlean, 2010). However, the majority of research tends to be from one methodological approach or the other. Evidence-based practice provides the scope to use studies from each paradigm to combine best clinical practice suggested by quantitative approaches with the insight and values of patients, clients, relatives and clinical staff as revealed by qualitative studies.

References

Holloway, I. and Wheeler, S. (2010) *Qualitative Research in Nursing and Healthcare*, 3rd edn. John Wiley & Sons, Chichester.

Houser, J. (2008) *Nursing Research: Reading, Using, and Creating Evidence*. Jones and Bartlett, Sudbury.

Polit, D. and Beck, C. (2008) *Nursing Research: Generating and Assessing Evidence for Nursing Practice*, 8th edn. Lippincott Williams & Wilkins, Philadelphia, PA.

Simons, L. and Lathlean, J. (2010) Mixed methods. In: K. Gerrish and A. Lacey (eds) *The Research Process in Nursing*, 6th edn, pp. 331–342. John Wiley & Sons, Chichester.

Tappen, R. (2011) *Advanced Nursing Research: From Theory to Practice*. Jones and Bartlett Learning, Sudbury.

For further resources for this chapter visit the companion website at
 www.wiley.com/go/glasper/nursingdissertation2e

Chapter 15

Chapter 16 **Using historical literature**

Diane Carpenter[1] and Alan Glasper[2]
[1]*University of Plymouth, UK*
[2]*University of Southampton, UK*

Scenario

In talking with the other students about her choice of topic for her dissertation, Sue mentioned that although she knew that larval therapy had been used in wound care in the past, she was a little unsure about when it had begun. Her interest had been aroused and she really wanted to investigate this in more detail. She was beginning to formulate some questions which she felt she would like to answer in order to place her topic in context. Also, she had experience of discussing this method of treatment with patients and receiving all sorts of reactions, many of which were negative. She had, she said, begun to wonder whether knowing more about its history might be useful to her in helping patients to accept it. She asked her student colleagues whether they thought that a historical investigation could ever be justified in modern healthcare. Sam raised the debate about different approaches to research and different types of evidence. 'In some areas', he said, 'randomised controlled trials are unsuitable. In many cases it would be unethical or impracticable to conduct them or there would be insufficient funding for a viable study'. Charlotte agreed and added that she supposed for that reason some areas of nursing were more inclined to use qualitative methods. She wondered whether historical research was qualitative. Alisha had read that it was often qualitative although there were examples of quantitative data being included, for example when studying the history of epidemics.

How to Write Your Nursing Dissertation, Second Edition.
Edited by Alan Glasper and Diane Carpenter.
© 2021 John Wiley & Sons Ltd. Published 2021 by John Wiley & Sons Ltd.
Companion website: www.wiley.com/go/glasper/nursingdissertation2e

Later that day Sue sat down to reflect on her conversation with Sam and wrote a list of questions that had occurred to her.

1. What is the use of history in a world focused on scientific evidence?
2. Where does historical research fit methodologically and is it rigorous?
3. Would such a study be considered primary research or would it be possible to appraise historical research that others had done?
4. Could I possibly justify doing a historical evidence-based practice project?
5. How would I go about undertaking a study based on historical evidence?

Sue posed these questions to her supervisor when she next saw her. She was told that the history department had a lecturer whose special interest was the history of health and social care. Sue made an appointment to see him and the following notes were taken from the answers she received.

What is the use of history in a world focused on scientific evidence?

John Tosh (2008:140–142) maintained that without the insights of applied history we are in danger of being 'unable to grasp how our world has come to be, or to detect the direction in which it is moving'. The principle of differentiating between past and present allows us to bring 'accumulated experience to bear on current problems'. If, for example, we did not take a patient's history and did not establish that they were allergic to penicillin, there could be dire consequences. Similarly, had we ignored the outcome of John Snow's epidemiological analysis of the source of cholera at the Broad Street pump in London, we might have been longer in preventing epidemics of it. Indeed, learning from history includes taking account of the cutting-edge science of an earlier time. Today's scientific research will be tomorrow's history. This does not mean that contemporary science is condemned to oblivion, rather that an understanding of the development of knowledge helps us to appreciate our current evidence base in context.

Should we find ourselves in the midst of a major disaster or in a remote place without recourse to medicines or equipment, knowledge of historical treatments might help prevent a fatality. For example, the ancient Greeks used reeds as catheters to empty bladders (Alexander *et al.*, 2006:872).

Where does historical research fit methodologically?

Polit and Beck (2006:216) define historical research as 'the systematic collection and critical evaluation of the data relating to past occurrences'. They

maintain that it relies largely on qualitative data. It can, however, make extensive use of quantitative data – in trawling through patient records to identify
demographic trends, for example. A historical enquiry is therefore likely to
unearth research which has used qualitative and/or quantitative data.
Historians are at odds about the extent to which they use theory in making
sense of their data. Although the past no longer exists, traces of it remain in
texts and artefacts. The researcher's task is to ascertain the truth of these as
far as he or she can deduce it (Berkhoffer, 2008:3–48). Some historical
researchers let this evidence speak for itself and conform to a purist empirical
approach. That is, they attempt to make sense of their research findings in
the context of what is already known about the period to which they are
thought to belong. Understanding the economic, political and social processes of the period in which the data were created helps to make sense of
them. Examples include the effects of the Industrial Revolution on city population size and spread of diseases such as cholera and typhoid.

A further illustration would be the way the prevailing social mores associated with class and sexual practices help us to understand the prevalence of
venereal disease. An example of failing to contextualise would be to criticise
the Victorians' treatment of women by today's standards rather than to
understand it in the context of the social attitudes, legislation and policy of
the time. Other researchers might see themselves as feminist, Marxist or
postmodern historians and would interpret their data according to their preferred paradigm or perspective. However, Bill McDowell (2002:13) cautioned
that studying the past according to preconceived theory was likely to produce
a 'disjointed and distorted account of past events'.

No matter which theoretical orientation is adopted, the historical research
method appears to be consistent and rigorous. Researchers:

1. identify the sources for their data;
2. authenticate their sources as genuine;
3. place their sources in the appropriate historical context;
4. interpret their findings;
5. place their research in relation to other work in the field (in historiographical context). [See E.H. Carr's (1990) and Geoffrey Elton's (1979) seminal
   works, as well as Mary Fulbrook's (2002) *Historical Theory* for further
   reading, as well as the section on appraisal of historical research.]

It is important, when considering the rigour of historical research to ascertain whether ethical approval was sought. There is a 100-year exclusion
period for access to medical records and a 30-year exclusion period for access
to official administrative records. Some older records might also be kept in
books that span several years and contain records within the exclusion

period. In such cases ethical approval is required. In all cases the archivists responsible for maintaining the records may still deny access to them. The researcher should give an account of any ethical issues associated with access to the data, including constraints of confidentiality for records accessed within the exclusion period. Medical records outside the exclusion period are within the public domain and names may be identified.

To ensure rigour, historians are expected to conform to a basic code of historical practice (Fulbrook, 2002:50). This requires commitment to basic honesty and integrity rather than deceit; absence of wilful distortions or omissions; commitment to accepting the possibility of revision of particular interpretations in the light of further evidence; and perhaps also (though this is less explicitly articulated by practising historians) commitment to enjoyment of the creativity of the historian as writer while still adhering to some notion of faithfulness to the past. It is unlikely, however, that this code could be determined when appraising historical research.

Would such a study constitute primary research or would it be possible to appraise historical research that others had done?

If you were to go to primary sources to undertake the historical method previously identified, then you would be engaged in primary research. This might be appropriate for a dissertation for a master's degree or for a PhD thesis. It is, however, possible to review and critically appraise the historical research published by others for an evidence-based practice project.

Polit and Beck (2006) corrected the myth that historical research does not create new knowledge and emphasised that it should not be confused with a literature review about historical events. In some instances historians find no relevant primary data upon which to draw. For example, many of Portsmouth's official records were destroyed by the bombing campaign of the Second World War. Under such circumstances, having demonstrated a concerted effort to trace sources and failing, researchers might use accounts made by others from, or about, the primary sources before they were lost. Such secondary accounts are different from literature reviews. In the former, the researcher aims to extrapolate the primary data and re-present or re-examine it; in the latter, he or she summarises what has been written about the topic broadly. A study of secondary sources will often require the researcher to reconsider the contextualisation and interpretations made earlier. As an example, in the nineteenth century patients in pauper lunatic asylums were often expected to work long days on the asylum farms or in the wards. Some researchers have condemned this as exploitative without considering what was normal for non-lunatic paupers at the time (Carpenter, 2010).

Could I possibly justify doing a historical evidence-based practice project?

Yes, and one example would be to explain current practice, for example the use of larval therapy in wound care. It might well be helpful to a patient disgusted with the idea of having live maggots applied to their wound, to understand how in the First World War it had saved the limbs and the lives of soldiers with compound fractures of the femur and other injuries.

In the same way, identifying the risk factors associated with patients with mental health problems absconding from hospital might result from an appraisal of the published work by those who analysed patient records, and critical incidents, dating back several years.

Finally, as a further illustration, reviewing the literature about oral history accounts of what made the greatest difference to grieving relatives might help the nurse prepare for that part of her role.

How do I go about undertaking a study based on historical evidence?

- Search for evidence in the usual way. Consider including a date range for the period in which you are interested.
- Consider grey literature. If your historical enquiry concerns fairly recent history you may find evidence in the form of old policies and procedures and older staff-members' memories. Care must be taken with the use of oral history, however, as memories can often become distorted over time.
- Select your literature as you would with any other evidence-based approach, that is, in terms of its relevance to your question and/or its closeness of fit to your patient group or clinical situation.
- Appraise the literature. You could use a broad qualitative framework (where this is appropriate) and/or apply the additional questions identified in Figure 16.1.
- Summarise your findings from this process and apply them to your clinical situation. You may compare historical approaches, practices, policies and guidelines with current versions, for example. Or you may try to create a timeline and outline change in practice over time. You should aim to answer the questions (i) what have I found and (ii) what is the relevance of this to contemporary practice?
- Disseminate your results. Take into account your target audience, for example patients, relatives or colleagues. Consider how you will present your findings. What do you hope the outcome will be? This may include policy change, or the creation of information leaflets, or an educational package as some examples. It may be appropriate to identify whether and how you will evaluate the effect or the effectiveness of sharing your results.

1	Was a research question or topic clearly identified?	Yes	No
2	Was a historical enquiry appropriate to answer the research question or address the topic?	Yes	No

3	Did the researcher identify his or her sources of data clearly?
	
	Did the researcher draw upon:
	   Primary sources (go to 3a)
	   Secondary sources (go to 3b)
	   Both primary and secondary sources (answer 3a and 3b)
		Yes	No

3a	Which primary data sources were used?
	
	Manuscript sources:
	   Administrative records
	   Clinical records
	   Minutes of meetings
	   Policies
	   Procedures
	   Other (state which)
	
	Contemporary published sources:
	   Books
	   Directories
	   Journal articles
	   Letters
	   Magazines and newspapers
	   Parliamentary papers
	   Public General Statutes
	   Other (state which)
		Yes	No

3b	Which secondary data sources were used?
	
	Published secondary sources:
	   Books
	   Journal articles
	
	Unpublished secondary sources:
	   Dissertations
	   Projects
	   Theses
	
	Electronic sources
	
	Other (state which)
		Yes	No

4	Were the sources authenticated? Did the researcher explain the provenance of the sources that were used? Hospital case books, for example, were usually clearly identified and often included an inserted label referring to relevant statutes that required them to be kept. Letters and diaries, however, are more easily faked	Yes	No
5	Was ethical approval necessary and sought?	Yes	No

Figure 16.1 Critical appraisal tool for historical research in health and social care. Sources: Carpenter (2010) and McDowell (2002).

6	Did the researcher use a particular paradigm or theoretical tradition with which to analyse/interpret the data? Was this clearly identified? Did the researcher justify his or her theoretical perspective? Were data interpreted consistently according to the chosen paradigm?	Yes	No
7	Were the findings analysed and interpreted appropriately? Did the researcher provide convincing arguments to support his or her interpretations? Were direct quotes from primary sources used to illustrate and support the data interpretation?	Yes	No
8	Did the researcher contextualise the findings? Did the researcher combine narrative (details of actual events) and analysis (placing the events in a broader social, economic or political context) sufficiently to support the conclusions? (McDowell, 2002:16–17)	Yes	No
9	Were the conclusions warranted by/consistent with the analysis and interpretation of the data? Were the conclusions believable? Did the researcher generalise his or her findings on the basis of the study? If so, was this justified? Was there a convincing argument based on consistent findings to suggest they could be generalised? NB: evidence for practice in one nineteenth-century hospital does not mean that every hospital practised in the same way. If, however, the researcher found similar accounts in a number of hospitals for the period, a generalised conclusion may be justified Did the researcher place his or her work with respect to any other eminent work in the field (in historiographical context)?	Yes	No

Figure 16.1 (Continued)

A week later the students met up again. Sue told them that she had determined to undertake a historical evidence-based practice project and felt confident she could justify doing it. She hoped that she would be able to use her findings to write an information leaflet for patients who were to be offered larval therapy. She believed that the historical information would help patients to see how the practice had changed over time but might also engage their interest and help alleviate their anxieties. Sam, Alisha and Charlotte were pleased Sue had decided on this course of action; Sam said he had met with James, a former colleague, who had made a study of shell shock and had offered his appraisal of an article he had found. He hoped it might be useful to her as a guide. The article James appraised was: May, C. (1998) Lord Moran's memoir: shell-shock and the pathology of fear, *Journal of the Royal Society of Medicine*, **91**, 95–100. His appraisal follows the approach of the tool in Figure 16.1.

1. This is a short essay without abstract but one which introduces its topic by reference to a case example taken from a primary source. The narrative clearly sets the scene for the article which the author confirms, a few paragraphs later, as having used the memoirs of Lord Moran (of the Royal Army Medical Corps during the First World War) to explore attitudes to shell shock. In so doing he reveals the tension between culpability and susceptibility and examines how this changed the definition of courage 'from individual acts of heroism to endurance in the face of random acts of annihilation' (p. 95).
2. Since the diagnosis of shell shock is synonymous with the Great War, a historical enquiry is entirely appropriate to its study.
3. (a) No manuscript sources were used but a discussion [James had] with the author revealed that these had been rigorously sought and were thought to have been destroyed during the Second World War. The author made use, therefore, of primary printed sources, including contemporary published books (amongst other things, Moran's diary memoirs) and journal articles, notably *The Lancet*. A War Office report of an enquiry into shell shock was a further source of data.
   (b) Whilst the study drew mainly upon primary published sources, it had recourse to more recent books and journal articles written by medical historians.
4. Since no manuscript sources were used authentication was not required.
5. Although this study was undertaken within the 100-year exclusion period, indeed 80 years from the end of the First World War, neither medical nor administrative documentary sources were available and therefore ethical approval was not required. None of the cases referred to from the published sources revealed the names of the sufferers and confidentiality was thereby sensitively maintained.
6. The researcher does not claim to have used any theoretical tradition with which he interpreted his findings. Rather, he appears to have used a purist empirical approach allowing the evidence to speak for itself.
7. The author has substantiated his assertions with reference to relevant primary sources, illustrated by appropriate and well-chosen direct quotes. He

has not claimed any unsupported outcomes from his analysis of the material.

8. Findings from the study have been contextualised clearly. One example is the description of the battlefield, the scale of advance and the effects of the resources of state and industry (p. 95). Another (p. 98) outlines issues of social class characteristic of later Edwardian Britain.

9. May identified change over time in attitudes towards shell shock. Since his main source, as the title suggests, was Lord Moran's memoirs, he has not attempted to generalise his findings, but used this case study to suggest attitudinal shift. However, he has not placed his contribution to the scholarship of this topic in historiographical context, despite referring to eminent historians of medical and psychiatric history such as Edward Shorter and Michael Stone.

James also commented that notwithstanding the emotive and evocative nature of the subject, there were no obvious distortions or omissions to embellish or minimise the findings. May's writing style demonstrates integrity, sensitivity and faithfulness to the past. He concluded his critique by affirming that the appraisal had supported confidence in the study's findings, which he would subsequently summarise and integrate into his own study. Having read through the article and James's critical appraisal of it, Sue felt more confident in attempting appraisals of the articles she had found and was eager to start the process.

References

Alexander, M.F., Fawcett, J.N. and Runciman, P. (eds) (2006) *Nursing Practice, Hospital and Home: The Adult.* Elsevier, London.

Berkhoffer, R.F. (2008) *Fashioning History: Current Practices and Principles.* Palgrave Macmillan, Basingstoke.

Carpenter, D.T. (2010) *Above all a patient should never be terrified: an examination of mental health care and treatment in Hampshire* 1845–1914. Unpublished PhD thesis, University of Portsmouth, UK.

Carr, E.H. (1990) *What Is History?*, 2nd edn. Penguin Books, London.

Elton, G.R. (1979) *The Practice of History, 9th impression.* Fontana, Sydney, Australia.

Fulbrook, M. (2002) *Historical Theory.* Routledge, London.

McDowell, W.H. (2002) *Historical Research: A Guide.* Longman, London.

May, C. (1998) Lord Moran's memoir: shell-shock and the pathology of fear. *Journal of the Royal Society of Medicine,* **91**, 95–100.

Polit, D.F. and Beck, C.T. (2006) *Essentials of Nursing Research: Methods, Appraisal, and Utilization,* 6th edn. Lippincott Williams & Wilkins, Philadelphia, PA.

Tosh, J. (2008) *Why History Matters.* Palgrave Macmillan, Basingstoke.

Further reading

Burnham, J.C. (2005) *What is Medical History?* Polity Press, Cambridge.

Lane, J. (2001) *A Social History of Medicine: Health, Healing and Disease in England,*
    1750–1950. Routledge, London.

Porter, R. (ed.) (2006) *Cambridge Illustrated History of Medicine*. Cambridge University
    Press, Cambridge.

For further resources for this chapter visit the companion website at
  www.wiley.com/go/glasper/nursingdissertation2e

Chapter 16

Section 5 **Critically appraising evidence**

Having collected some relevant research articles, the students are faced with selecting appropriate critical appraisal tools to evaluate their selected papers. Sam has been advised to use Parahoo's critiquing approach, Sue and Charlotte find the Critical Appraisal Skills Programme (CASP) tools useful and Alisha also finds Greenhalgh's (2019) range of appraisal tools very helpful.

Chapter 17 Selecting and using appraisal tools: how to interrogate research papers

Diane Carpenter[1] and Alan Glasper[2]
[1]*University of Plymouth, UK*
[2]*University of Southampton, UK*

> **Scenario**
>
> All the students have spent time in the library and have conducted a full search of the bibliographical databases. They have also perused the grey literature and have conduced hand searches of archived journals. After applying inclusion and exclusion criteria they have sourced some relevant data-driven research articles and retrieved them. All need to select an appropriate critical appraisal tool to evaluate and appraise their selected papers. They know that the critical appraisal needs to be a component of the evidence-based practice healthcare dissertation/final project or evidence-informed decision-making assignment as it is an important aspect of understanding the evidence base for practice. Now they must make sure they get the best from each article and convey their knowledge using a critical analysis style of writing.

Introduction

This chapter is designed to help students who are writing an evidence-based practice healthcare dissertation/final project or evidence-informed decision-making assignment to fully comprehend the process of critiquing empirical journal papers. In this chapter a range of critiquing models are discussed and, furthermore, in other separate chapters how these models can be used to critique individual papers is described.

This chapter is based on an earlier chapter by Alan Glasper and Colin Rees.

How to Write Your Nursing Dissertation, Second Edition.
Edited by Alan Glasper and Diane Carpenter.
© 2021 John Wiley & Sons Ltd. Published 2021 by John Wiley & Sons Ltd.
Companion website: www.wiley.com/go/glasper/nursingdissertation2e

What is critical appraisal? What are critical appraisal tools? Why is critical appraisal of published research important? What does critical appraisal mean to nurses and other healthcare professionals?

Burls (2009) suggests that critical appraisal is the process of carefully and systematically examining research to judge its trustworthiness, value and relevance in a particular context. Critical appraisal is a process to be learned by healthcare practitioners to enable them to evaluate not only what an article says but also the quality of the research that has produced it. Poor research will not produce reliable results. By following a systematic process, a professional can weigh up its value and relevance for their own area of practice, usually in a clinical domain. Thus, academic critiquing is an essential skill that nurses and others need if they are to use research evidence in contemporary healthcare. These skills facilitate finding and using appropriate research evidence reliably and efficiently in practice.

Critical appraisal of published research papers is a process that any healthcare professional faced with solving a clinical problem must undertake before attempting to make any change in practice. The method through which healthcare professionals critically evaluate published empirical papers is one which allows the practitioner to make a sound evaluation of the worth and provenance of the material reported in specific journals. In identifying the strengths and weaknesses of the published paper, the practitioner can make a value judgement of the worth of the reported findings and make a decision about its applicability to their own area of practice. The systematic appraisal of papers using a recognised appraisal tool allows the practitioner to make reliable conclusions about the value of the work they are reading and make assessments as to the relevance of the data to their own arena of practice and, importantly, judge if applying the evidence might make a difference to patient outcomes.

If nurses and other healthcare professionals decide and plan to make changes to patient care management, they need to be able to:

- decide if the research being reported has been conducted in such a way to ensure that the finding is both valid and reliable;
- be able to understand and make sense of the results;
- decide if the research is strong enough to suggest changes to practice.

There are many different critiquing tools available: some target specific types of study (e.g. qualitative) and some are generic and can be used to appraise any paper. Katrak *et al.* (2004) have shown that there are no tools that are a bespoke fit to healthcare research and that the interpretation nurses make after a critical appraisal of an individual research paper needs to be considered in light of the individual critical appraisal tool which has been used.

What is the best critical appraisal tool to use?

It is beyond the scope of this chapter to discuss the full range of critiquing tools available. Most of them are very similar and all are intended to help readers more fully understand the various elements of published empirical papers. Some, such as CASP, have been designed specifically for certain types of paper, for example randomised controlled trials. The University of South Australia International Centre for Allied Health Evidence (https://www.unisa.edu.au/research/Health-Research/Research/Allied-Health-Evidence/Resources/) offers a full and comprehensive discussion of the attributes of many popular healthcare critiquing tools. Additionally, the Scottish Intercollegiate Guidelines Network (SIGN) has developed evidence-based clinical practice guidelines for the NHS (https://www.sign.ac.uk/what-we-do/methodology/checklists/).

All healthcare professionals need to develop the skills of critiquing research-based papers. Critical appraisal is the systematic and unbiased detailed examination of all the reported elements of a published paper or study to allow judgement of both the merits or strengths and the weakness or limitations in order to facilitate both the meaning and relevance to practice (Burns and Grove, 2009).

Many professionals when they first encounter the term 'critique' mistakenly think of the verb 'to criticise', but in this context the word has a different meaning. A critique is a constructive evaluation of a piece of published work which is intended to be objective, unbiased and impartial, taking a balanced view of both the content of the paper and of the research process which has been used by the author(s).

Critiquing is a skill that requires practice. Although many critiquing tools are available, this chapter considers critiquing tools which have been developed by:

1. Crombie
2. CASP
3. Parahoo
4. Rees.

Some critiquing tools have been designed for analysing different types of research approaches. For example, CASP has a whole suite of critiquing tools and Rees has developed a tool for the analysis of both qualitative and quantitative papers, whereas Crombie and Parahoo have developed one model which can be applied to all types of published research. Chapters 18–20 show in detail how these tools (namely CASP and Parahoo) can be applied to specific types of research papers.

Commencing your critique

Before making your final selection of papers to critique it is useful to consider McCarthy and O'Sullivan (2008), who suggest that the first priority when considering applying the critiquing process is to consider if an individual paper is worth reading. How can we do this? The following are questions that will help.

- Is from a peer-reviewed journal? This will help indicate if the paper is from a reliable source, such as a well-known professional nursing journal. This can be easily verified by going online to the journal webpages, where full details of how papers are selected for publication should give details of the peer review process.
- Consider the title and whether it is relevant to the topic you are exploring. What does it say? Can you trust it? And will it contribute to your practice?

This process will allow you to develop a 'long shortlist' of suitable papers that you will consider before making your final short list to engage in the full critiquing review process (Box 17.1). The shortlist of papers should be clearly indicated in a table at the beginning of the critiquing chapter if your dissertation requires this.

Box 17.1   How many papers should be critiqued for an evidence-based practice healthcare dissertation/final project or evidence-informed decision-making assignment?

This will vary from university to university but typically there is an expectation that the student will use a minimum of three where there is a paucity of published papers up to a maximum of five where there is a significant body of knowledge available (more for a master's degree). This is where the student can develop a long shortlist of papers before making a final selection of those papers that best fit the PICO/SPICE or similar question posed and meet the full inclusion and exclusion criteria which have been set.

   For MSc dissertations in some universities up to 14 papers may be critiqued to ascertain answers to more complex clinical questions; for a PhD a full appraisal of all pertinent literature is expected.

Is an individual paper worth adding to the shortlist? Preparing your initial long shortlist

When faced with a choice of papers, the task is to narrow the field to whatever number the university prescribes in its student assignment guidelines. In making an informed decision to prepare a long shortlist selection you will find it helpful to read the description of what the author(s) examined in the paper and answer these questions.

1. How do they justify the need for the study?
2. How did they carry out the study?
3. What did they find?
4. What did they conclude?
5. Assess if rigour has been applied to the research process – how well was it thought through and what steps were taken to reduce problems of bias, reliability and validity?
6. What is the study's contribution to your professional practice? For example, does it provide clear evidence for continuing, adapting or challenging practice? Who might benefit from the study, and in what way?

Now make your final shortlist selection (consider putting this in a table format).

Commencing your initial read and review of an empirical journal paper

Before you start, and irrespective of the particular critiquing model you have selected for your own evidence-based practice healthcare dissertation/final project or evidence-informed decision-making assignment, there are a number of elements that should be considered when critically reviewing a paper. Firstly, reading empirical or data-driven research papers is very different from reading a newspaper or a holiday novel. This type of reading is active rather than passive, requiring significant concentration and the burning of many calories by the cognitive centres of the brain! This type of reading requires an active, analytical and reflective approach (Table 17.1). To hone these active reading and analytical skills it is necessary to divide the paper into its constituent parts. Many journal papers are already structured in this way to make their reading more focused. Every editor of every health professional journal knows that their readers are busy practitioners with limited time to read. This is why most good journal papers will include a detailed abstract informing the reader of the banner headlines of the study contained within the published paper. Many busy practitioners will only

Table 17.1 Stages in critical reading of research articles.

Stage	Purpose	Activities or critical questions:
Preliminary understanding (skim or speed read)	Skimming or speed-reading to gain understanding of the content and layout of the paper	• Use a highlighter pen to show the main steps in the research process • Make notes (comments and questions) • Note down key variables • Highlight new or unfamiliar terms and significant sentences • Look up unfamiliar terms and write in definitions
Comprehensive understanding	Increasing understanding of concepts and research terms	• Review all unfamiliar terms before second reading • Clarify any additional terms • Read additional sources as necessary • Identify how the main concepts relate to each other and the context of the study • Write brief summary of the main idea or themes of the article in your own words • Identify any further questions or areas that need further clarification
Analysis understanding (breaking into parts)	Break the study into parts; understand each aspect of the study. Relate to steps in the research process. At this point you can start to critique the study using a critiquing framework or criteria, applying them to each step in the research process	• What is the purpose of this article? • Am I clear about the specific design used, so I can apply appropriate critiquing criteria? • How are the major parts of the article related to the research process? • How was the study carried out? Can I explain it step by step? • What are the researchers' main conclusions? • Can I say I understand the parts of the article and summarise them in my own words?
Synthesis understanding	Pulling the above steps together to make a (new) whole, making sense of it and explaining relationships	• Review notes on how each step compared with the critiquing criteria • Briefly summarise the study in your own words, identifying the main components, and the overall strengths and weaknesses • This is a critical commentary on the study rather than a description or précis of it

Source: LoBiondo-Wood *et al.* (2002). Reproduced with permission of Elsevier. © 2002, Elsevier.

ever get round to reading the abstract but for the purposes of undertaking an evidence-based practice project as part of a university course or as part of professional development it is necessary to drill deeper into the hidden recesses of the paper.

Detailed and methodical reading will help the reader initially gain an outline of the research, and facilitate an understanding of how the various parts of the paper fit together. To become an active reader certain questions need to be asked, which in turn generate answers that help in the decision-making process of assessing the relative value of the paper to one's own field of practice. The various critiquing tools available for practitioners to use provide such a question framework.

Points to consider about the paper(s) before using any critiquing tool

Focus

This is the first aspect to be considered when starting to read a paper, as this allows the reader to put it in the context of existing knowledge about the subject. This is usually stated in the opening paragraph or separately as simply words, concepts or variables covered in the article. Often the title of the paper conveys at least some of this but cannot be relied upon to do so. *Here, you as the reader are making a judgement about the sphere of the paper content.*

Background

The abstract and opening paragraphs should convey the background to the study and readers should expect to see citable evidence as to why the particular topic is a problem worthy of investigation (e.g. pain relief after spinal surgery or larvae therapy to promote wound healing). Most studies should begin with a definition or an identification of the practice area problem and this will be followed by a broad review of the contemporary literature pertinent to the subject. *Readers should expect the authors to be critical in their own appraisal of the literature being reviewed!* Importantly, use this to identify the strengths and weaknesses of previous studies to illuminate the reasons why the current study has been undertaken and reported. In this section of the paper authors will present the overall framework of the study.

Study aims, hypothesis or objectives

These should be clearly stated and should emerge after reading the initial part of the paper. Usually the aim/hypothesis or objectives will be cited first in the abstract and then more comprehensively described within the body of the paper.

Chapter 17

Methodology

This section should be simply stated in the abstract, and then in more detail under a heading of method/methodology. This aspect of the paper should identify the research design of the project. The research design should be appropriate to the research question. Some research questions will require a qualitative approach, for example patients' perceptions of ambulatory day-care surgery versus inpatient care. Others may require a quantitative approach, for example the effect of gentle exercise on blood pressure measurement in the elderly. Irrespective of the design, the authors of the paper should give sufficient detail of the methods they have used to elicit data to answer the original research question or topic area they have posed. Authors should acknowledge both the strengths and weaknesses of the data collection tool and give details of any other data collection method they might have used in endeavouring to triangulate their data, that is, look at the topic using more than one data collection tool to ensure the accuracy of the results.

Good papers will also in the method section give detail of any pilot work undertaken as part of the study. This helps to strengthen the validity of the research tools they have used, for example all questionnaires should be piloted.

Scenario

What nurses say and do about healthy eating: using triangulation to support or reject study findings

Sam has been chatting to one of his postgraduate colleagues who is a senior health visitor undertaking a taught Doctorate in Clinical Practice. She has used a quantitative survey questionnaire in an attempt to measure lifestyles of a cohort of student nurses and, in particular, what they eat. Additionally, to help triangulate or corroborate her findings she has interviewed a subgroup of the cohort using a qualitative semi-structured interview schedule. Surprisingly, what she found was that rather than confirm the veracity of the survey instrument findings, the student nurses at interview demonstrated that what they said in the survey and what they actually did was very different. Hence, the sample of nurses revealed, at interview, that they were drinking more alcohol, smoking more cigarettes and eating more high-fat content ready meals than they had admitted to in the survey.

Ethical considerations

All reported studies published in journals should acknowledge the ethical issues related to, among others, consent in the study. The reader of the paper should be able to ascertain that the researcher(s) have gained ethical approval.

Main findings

All published studies should give clear details of the main findings of the research, either qualitative or quantitative. How the results are displayed is also important. It is very important to note that it is not expected that the authors of the papers will define and explain the statistical terms they have used; it is assumed that readers will be familiar with the various tests used by the researchers. Practitioners initially find the world of healthcare statistics a minefield of confusing numbers, symbols and words.

Discussion

Following the results section all journal papers should discuss the issues that have arisen from the findings. Additionally, the researchers should comment on any limitations to the study, for example small sample size or poor response rate to a questionnaire. It is also usual for papers to cite the findings of other similar studies to compare or contrast the findings with their own.

Conclusion

Published papers should always include a conclusion in which the authors briefly sum up their findings and, importantly, the implications, if any, for practice.

Applying a critiquing framework tool of your choice to your selected papers

> **Scenario**
>
> The students have been advised to visit the local supermarket to purchase a large pack of children's highlighter pens. Sue and Charlotte have also acquired some exotic fluorescent colours, which they believe will be useful because they now have a different colour for each of the critiquing tool questions. Their idea comes from the work of Riley (1996) who used this as a method of identifying commonalities in transcribed qualitative interviews. Sue has selected four papers for her critiquing exercise. Sam and she joke about the cutting up of the papers colour by colour to facilitate answering the critiquing tool questions across all the selected papers, but Charlotte actually intends to do this. Alisha is also like-minded!

Tasks to do before commencing a full critique of a selection of journal papers

Having made your final choice of papers and before you begin the task of critiquing, it is important to first do the following.

1. Buy a large pack of colour highlighter pens. These can be obtained in most supermarkets and are invaluable in the critiquing process.
2. Have at least three or four copies of each your selected papers: one to carry with you in your handbag, briefcase or rucksack to read on the bus, train or plane or in your coffee break; one to identify specific details using the colour highlighter pens. (Some students like to cut up one copy of the papers with scissors after highlighting and reassemble piece by piece to match the criteria of the specific critiquing tool they are using.) Finally, keep a spare copy for insurance – just in case!

Using Savage and Callery grids to undertake a preliminary critique

Savage and Callery (2000) used specially designed grids (Figure 17.1) to highlight the primary attributes of the papers they critiqued in their literature review of parental participation in the care of their children in hospital. Some students who are writing evidence-based practice healthcare dissertation/final project or evidence-informed decision-making assignment find this process helpful as a first stage in their critique of the papers they have selected following their search of the literature. After completion, some students find it particularly helpful to print these grids in landscape and on

Author (year) Country	Aim(s) of study	Methodological Issues		Relevant/ key findings
		Sample	Design, data collection and analysis, rigour/ reliability and validity	

Figure 17.1 Savage and Callery grid.

Activity 17.1

Source the chapter below from the Glasper and Ireland textbook (most academic libraries will have a copy):

  Savage, E. and Callery, P. (2000) Parental participation in the care of hospitalised children: a review of the research evidence. In: E.A. Glasper and L. Ireland (eds) *Evidence-based Child Health Care Challenges for Practice*, pp. 67–89. Macmillan, Basingstoke, UK.

  Discuss in your learning group how Savage and Callery used a grid to display the primary attributes of the research literature on parental participation.

Chapter 17

oversize paper (A2), which they then stick on a wall next to their computers. This helps them to see the primary features of all the papers they have selected for critiquing.

Remember, before wring your critiquing chapter you should have a short introduction informing the reader which papers you are critiquing as well as an outline of the critiquing framework you have selected.

Critiquing models

The Crombie model of critiquing

Crombie's (1996) concise guide to critical appraisal has been published by the *British Medical Journal* and is a very useful model to use in understanding the process of critical appraisal of health research. Many practitioners, such as nurses, find it helpful to follow Crombie's framework to help them think about the process of critiquing a research paper (qualitative or quantitative).

1. Why was it done? (Objectives)
   (a) What was the rationale for undertaking this study?
   (b) What was the purpose of the study?
   (c) Was the research question clearly stated?
2. How was it done? (Methods)
   (a) Was the research design appropriate to address the research question?
   (b) How was the sample selected?
   (c) How were the data collected?
   (d) How were the data analysed?
   (e) Were ethical issues discussed?

3. What has it found? (Results)
   (a) Are the findings clearly presented?
   (b) Do the findings answer the research question?
4. What are the implications? (Conclusions)
   (a) Were the findings discussed?
   (b) Are implications for future practice summarised?

The CASP models of critiquing

The Critical Appraisal Skills Programme (CASP) has been designed by Solutions For Public Health (http://www.sph.nhs.uk/what-we-do/public-health-workforce/resources/critical-appraisals-skills-programme) and provides seven different critiquing tools, each designed for different types of study and these are freely available to download from the website. Given the complexity of this suite of tools only two exemplars will be discussed here.

1. Making sense of randomised controlled trials.
2. Making sense of qualitative research.

Each of these tools has been used within this book to critique papers: Chapter 19 uses tool (1) to dissect a randomised controlled trial paper and Chapter 18 uses tool (2) to dissect a qualitative paper.

10 questions to help you make sense of randomised controlled trials
Although this CASP tool poses 10 questions, each question is further subdivided and the full tool with all the sub-questions is available through the website to this book at www.wiley.com/go/glasper/nursingdissertation2e.

1. Did the study ask a clearly focused question?
2. Was this a randomised controlled trial and was it appropriately so? (Is it worth continuing to read the paper?)
3. Were the participants appropriately allocated to intervention and control groups?
4. Were participants, staff and study personnel 'blind' to participants' study group?
5. Were all participants who entered the trial accounted for at its conclusion?
6. Were the participants in all groups followed up and data collected in the same way?
7. Did the study have enough participants to minimise the play of chance?
8. How are the results presented and what is the main result?
9. How precise are the results?
10. Were all the important outcomes considered so the results can be applied?

These questions are further subdivided and a full example of a critique of a paper using this model can be found in Chapter 19.

10 questions to help you make sense of qualitative research
Although this CASP tool designed to critique qualitative research papers poses 10 questions, each question is further subdivided and the full tool with all the sub-questions is available through the website to this book at www. wiley.com/go/glasper/nursingdissertation2e.

1. Was there a clear statement of the aims of the research?
2. Is a qualitative methodology appropriate? (Is it worth continuing?)
3. Was the research design appropriate to address the aims of the research?
4. Was the recruitment strategy appropriate to the aims of the research?
5. Were data collected in a way that addressed the research issue?
6. Has the relationship between researcher and participants been adequately considered?
7. Have ethical issues been taken into consideration?
8. Was the data analysis sufficiently rigorous?
9. Is there a clear statement of findings?
10. How valuable is the research?

The Parahoo model of critiquing
Parahoo (1997) suggests asking the questions identified in the following sections when undertaking a critique of any research paper, qualitative or quantitative. These questions are further subdivided and a full example of a critique of a paper using this model can be found in Chapter 18.

The Parahoo framework consists of the following headings that are based on the structure most often used to report quantitative studies in research journals, although this model can be applied to qualitative studies. (An electronic copy of this model can also be downloaded from the companion website to this book at www.wiley.com/go/glasper/nursingdissertation2e.) The  headings are as follows.

- Title of study
- Abstract
- Literature review/Background
- Methodology or Design
- Results
- Discussion and interpretation (including limitations)
- Recommendations

Chapter 17

Title of study
Does the title convey the study clearly and accurately?

Abstract
Does the abstract give a short and concise summary of the following aspects of the study?

- Background
- Aim
- Designs
- Results
- Conclusions

Literature review/Background
- Is the importance of study justified?
- What is the context of this study?
- Does the literature review show the gaps in knowledge which this study seeks to fill?

Aims/objectives/research questions/hypotheses
- Are the aims of the study clear?

Design of study
- What is the design of the study? Is it the most appropriate for the aims of the study?
- Are the main concepts (to be measured) defined?
- What are the methods of data collection? Are they constructed for the purpose of the current study or do the researchers use existing ones?
- Who collected data? Can this introduce bias in the study?
- In studies where there are more than one group, is there a description of what intervention/treatment each group receives?
- Is the setting where the study is carried out adequately described?
- Who was selected? From what population were they selected? What was the precise method of selection and allocation? Was there a sample size calculation?
- Was ethical approval obtained? Are there any other ethical implications?

Data analysis
- Was there a separate section in the paper that explained the planned analyses prior to the presentation of the results?
- Which statistical methods were relied on?
- Is it clear how the statistical tests were applied to the data and groups?

Results
- Are the results clearly presented?
- Are the results for all the aims presented?
- Are the results fully presented?

Discussion
- Is it a balanced discussion? Have all possible explanations for the results been given?
- Are the results discussed in the context of previous studies?
- Are the results fully discussed?
- Are the limitations of the study discussed?

Conclusions/Recommendations
- Are the conclusions justified?
- Are there recommendations for policy, practice or further research?
- Are the results/conclusions helpful for my practice?
- Are the results generalisable?

Funding
- Is there potential conflict of interest (if information on funding is provided)?

The Rees (2011) model for critiquing quantitative research

An example of a critique using the Rees model for a quantitative study can be found in Chapter 19. (An electronic copy of this model can also be downloaded from the companion website to this book at www.wiley.com/go/glasper/nursingdissertation2e.)

Focus
In broad terms, what is the theme of the article? What are the key words you would file this under? Is the title a clue to the focus? How important is this for the profession/practice?

Background
What argument or evidence does the researcher provide to suggest this topic is worthwhile exploring? Is there a review of previous literature on the subject, or reference to government or professional reports that illustrate its importance? Are gaps in the literature or inadequacies with previous methods highlighted? Are local problems or changes that justify the study presented? Is there a trigger that answers the question 'Why did they do it then?'. Is there a theoretical or conceptual framework that helps us to see how all the elements in the study may be related?

Aim
What is the aim of the research? This will usually start with the word 'to', for example 'the aim of this research was *to examine/determine/compare/establish*, etc.' If relevant, is there a hypothesis? If there is, what are the dependent and independent variables? Are there concept and operational definitions for the key concepts?

Study design
What is the broad research approach? Is it quantitative or qualitative? Is the design experimental, descriptive or correlational? Is the study design appropriate to the terms of reference?

Data collection method
Which tool of data collection has been used? Has a single method been used or triangulation? Has the author addressed the issues of reliability and validity? Has a pilot study been conducted or tool used from previous studies? Have any limitations of the tool been recognised?

Ethical considerations
Were the issues of informed consent and confidentiality addressed? Was any harm or discomfort to individuals balanced against any benefits? Did an ethics committee approve the study?

Sample
Who or what makes up the sample? Are there clear inclusion and exclusion criteria? What method of sampling was used? Are those in the sample typical and representative of the larger group, or are there any obvious elements of bias? On how many people/things/events are the results based?

Data presentation
In what form are the results presented: tables, bar graphs, pie charts, raw figures or percentages? Does the author explain and comment on these? Has the author used correlation to establish whether certain variables are associated with each other? Have tests of significance been used to establish to what extent any differences between groups/variables could have happened by chance? Can you make sense of the way the results have been presented or could the author have provided more explanation?

Main findings
Which are the most important results that relate to the aim? (Think of this as putting the results in priority order – which is the most important result followed by the next most important result, and so on. There may only be a small number of these.)

Conclusion and recommendations

Using the author's own words, what is the answer to the aim? If relevant, is the hypothesis accepted or rejected? Are the conclusions based on, and supported by, the results? What recommendations are made for practice? Are these relevant, specific and feasible?

Readability

How readable is it? Is it written in a clear interesting style or is it heavy going? Does it assume a lot of technical knowledge about the subject and/or research procedures (i.e. is there much unexplained jargon)?

Practice implications

Once you have read it, what is the answer to the question 'so what?' Was it worth doing and publishing? How could it be related to practice? Who might find it relevant and in what way? What questions does it raise for practice and further study?

The Rees (2011) model for critiquing qualitative research

Focus

What is the key issue, concept or problem the work examines? What are the key words you would file this article under? Are there clues to the focus in title? How important is this for practice and the profession? Is the type of qualitative design included in the title?

Background

What argument or evidence does the researcher provide for exploring this issue, concept or problem? Is there a review of previous literature on the subject or reference to government or professional reports that illustrate its importance? Are gaps in the literature or inadequacies with previous methods highlighted? Does the literature review examine the concepts or issues that form the focus? Is there an attempt to justify the study within the context of a qualitative research design? If this is grounded theory, there may not be a comprehensive review of the literature at this point, although some reference to previous work may be included as an illustration of its importance. There should be some argument or background information to justify looking at this particular subject.

Aim

What is the stated aim of the research? This will usually start with the word 'to'. There will not be a hypothesis or the identification of dependent and independent variables, as qualitative research answers a level 1 question. There may be an attempt to provide a definition for the concept that forms the focus of the study. On the whole you will find the aim very broad and general and not as detailed as in quantitative research.

Study design
There may be an acknowledgement that the study is qualitative in design and then the type of method specified. The main alternatives are as follows.

1. *Phenomenological*: explores what it is like to have a certain experience, such as a delivery, a pregnancy or threatened miscarriage, and how people interpret that experience.
2. *Ethnographic*: the researcher enters and participates in the world of the subject by listening, observing and asking questions in order to understand their view of the world.
3. *Grounded theory*: identifies concepts which arise from the analysis of the data collected and may also suggest a theory or hypothesis that explains or predicts some of the behaviour that has emerged in the study.

It is important that the philosophy behind the method suits the intentions of the research.

Tool of data collection
Here we are interested not only in the technique used to collect the information but also in the amount of detail available on the circumstances under which the data were collected. This contributes to the credibility of the study. This should include details of the environment in which the data were collected, over what period of time data collection took place, and any other details that allow us to visualise the conduct of data collection. Did the researcher spend sufficient time, either in observing the life and behaviour of the subjects, or in interviewing subjects, to produce sufficient depth to the data? Because of the flexible way that data are gathered and the way the method will change during data collection, a pilot study will not usually be employed. However, the researcher should include details of how they have attempted to achieve procedural rigour in the way the study was conducted. Did they check with those in the study that the information collected was accurate (members' check)?

Ethical considerations
As with qualitative studies, it is important that the researcher has protected the participant from harm and has gained informed consent from those taking part in the study. It should not be possible to identify individuals or places where the study took place where this might affect anonymity. The researcher should illustrate ethical rigour, including, where appropriate, approach to a

local research ethics committee (LREC), or in American studies an institutional review board (IRB), to approve the research.

Sample

Who forms the sample and what are their basic characteristics? The sample size may be quite small, even down to three or four, but more usually about 10–15. This may be dictated by theoretical saturation, that is, data collection stops once no new themes or categories emerge from the analysis. In qualitative research it is important to assess whether the participants possess the relevant knowledge or carry out the activity in which the researcher is interested. Has the researcher demonstrated that the participants are able to provide relevant information and are not open to any kind of bias? The reader must consider to what extent the findings, theory or conceptual categories may apply to other settings. This contributes to its *fittingness* to be applied elsewhere.

Data presentation

The data will be presented in the form of description, dialogue or comments from participants. Is this '*thick*' and '*rich*' description? Is there sufficient detail for us to almost feel that we are there? Do the quotes from participants clearly illustrate the concepts they are being used to illustrate? Is there overdependence on comments from a small number of the participants in the sample? Has the researcher detailed how they ensured that the data were accurately recorded and representative of the data gathered? Is there anything about the circumstances in which the data were collected that could have threatened the accuracy of the data? Is it possible to discover the *decision trail* used by the researcher to determine how the raw data was processed into the categories presented in the results section? This contributes to its *auditability*. Given the same data, it should be possible, following the decision trail, to arrive at similar categories and conclusions. Does the researcher present the findings in the participants' own words rather than reinterpreting what was said or done?

Main findings

What are the key concepts or categories developed from the data? Do the concepts and categories presented cover all the data gathered? Were the findings checked either by the participants (members' check) or examined by other experts in the field (*peer review*)? Are the main findings credible, that is, have attempts been made to support the accuracy of the results through rigour in the way in which the study was conducted? Does the researcher discuss the findings and relate these to the literature, or do they leave the quotes to speak for themselves?

Conclusion

Is there a clear answer to the aim? Does the researcher propose a relationship between the concepts and categories developed in the analysis to form a clear conceptual or theoretical framework? Does the conceptual or theoretical framework reflect the data? Has the conclusion been arrived at inductively (built up from the findings)?

Readability

Does the researcher present the description of the social circumstances described in the research in sufficient detail that one can almost imagine being there, and hear the participants talking and carrying out the activities described? Is it possible to recognise the concepts described as related to practical experience? Is the report written in a simple and understandable way? Is there a clear 'story line' emerging from the research?

Relevance to practice

Are the findings relevant to practice or professional knowledge? Is it an important area related to current concerns and issues within the profession? Does the research satisfy the criteria of *transferability*, that is, can the findings in the form of the theory, concepts or categories developed through the study be applied to other situations, or are they only applicable to the place and the people where the study took place? Do you feel the research has sensitised you to issues or provided further insight? Has it confirmed views you might have already held?

Scenario

Sam, Alisha and Charlotte have decided to use Parahoo's critiquing approach, whereas Sue has been advised to use the Rees model. All the students are aware that all the critiquing tools, at some point in the exercise, ask for a consideration of the results section of the papers. Depending on the level of the course – foundation degree, undergraduate or postgraduate – the amount of information concerning statistical information will vary but, for all evidence-based practice healthcare dissertations/final projects or evidence-informed decision-making assignments, at least a preliminary understanding of the tests used by the researchers is recommended.

Conclusion

This chapter has endeavoured to give an overview of the process of critiquing research papers and has sought to outline a number of critiquing models used in the appraisal of contemporary healthcare literature. Note that in Chapter 16, the authors provide details of how historical literature can be appraised.

Scenario

The students have completed the critiquing of their selected papers. They are now in the final stages of their evidence-based practice healthcare dissertation/final project or evidence-informed decision-making assignment and are planning to write a short section summing up the relative strengths and weaknesses of the papers they have read and comprehensively critiqued. They have all been advised to include within this section a table showing what these are (Figure 17.2).

Study	Strengths	Limitations	
1			
2			
3			
4			

Figure 17.2 Strengths and limitations resulting from the critiquing process. (Example of blank table for your use. A copy can also be downloaded from the companion website at www.wiley.com/go/glasper/nursingdissertation2e).

References

Burls, A. (2009) What is critical appraisal? www.whatisseries.co.uk (accessed 26 May 2012).

Burns, N. and Grove, S. (2009) *The Practice of Nursing Research: Appraisal, Synthesis, and Generation of Evidence*, 6th edn. Saunders, St. Louis, MO.

Crombie, I. (1996) *The Pocket Guide to Critical Appraisal*. BMJ Publications, London.

Greenhalgh, T. (2019) *How to Read a Paper*, 6th edn. Blackwell Publishing, Oxford.

Katrak, P., Bialocerkowski, A.E., Massy-Westropp, S. *et al.* (2004) A systematic review of the content of critical appraisal tools. BMC Medical Research Methodology, **4**, 22.

LoBiondo-Wood, G., Haber, J. and Krainovich-Miller, B. (2002) Critical reading strategies: overview of the research process. In: G. LoBiondo-Wood and J. Haber (eds) *Nursing Research: Methods, Critical Appraisal, and Utilization*, 5th edn, chapter 2. Mosby, St. Louis, MO.

McCarthy, G. and O'Sullivan, D. (2008) Evaluating the literature. In: R. Watson, H. McKenna, S. Cowman and J. Keady (eds) *Nursing Research: Designs and Methods*, pp. 113–123. Churchill Livingstone, Edinburgh.

Parahoo, K. (1997) *Nursing Research: Principles, Process and Issues*. Macmillan, Basingstoke, UK.

Rees, C. (2011) *Introduction to Research for Midwives*, 3rd edn. Churchill Livingstone, Edinburgh.

Riley, J. (1996) *Getting the Most from Your Data. A Handbook of Practical Ideas on How to Analyse Qualitative Data*. Technical and Educational Services Ltd.

Savage, E. and Callery, P. (2000) Parental participation in the care of hospitalised children: a review of the research evidence. In: A.E. Glasper and L. Ireland (eds) *Evidence-based Child Health Care Challenges for Practice*, pp. 67–89. Macmillan, Basingstoke, UK.

For further resources for this chapter visit the companion website at

☉ **www.wiley.com/go/glasper/nursingdissertation2e**

Chapter 18 Critically reviewing qualitative papers using a CASP critiquing tool

Diane Carpenter[1] and Alan Glasper[2]
[1]*University of Plymouth, UK*
[2]*University of Southampton, UK*

Scenario

Sue, the top-up degree student, and Sam, the MSc student, have identified a range of qualitative papers that they need to critically appraise as part of their dissertations. Meanwhile Charlotte and Alisha have both received feedback in earlier essays that higher marks can be achieved when students comment on the nature and strength of evidence to support their discussion points and they have both found qualitative research articles they wish to refer to in their final assignments. The four students meet at a drop-in workshop session at their university library aimed at helping them develop their skills of critical appraisal. As they have all found qualitative papers to critique they have been advised to use the Critical Appraisal Skills Programme (CASP, 2018) appraisal checklist for qualitative research.

The tool designed to make sense of qualitative evidence has been developed for those who are not very confident or familiar with qualitative research and, as such, provides a starting point. The appraisal tool is copyright protected but it may be used by individuals so long as it is appropriately referenced; the complete tool can be found at https://casp-uk.net/wp-content/uploads/2018/01/CASP-Qualitative-Checklist-2018.pdf and more details about CASP can be found at https://casp-uk.net/. All the students attending the seminar to help with their critical appraisal skills for qualitative research have been given an article to appraise. The article's title is 'Sick children's perceptions of clown doctor humour' and was written by Katy Weaver, Gill

---

How to Write Your Nursing Dissertation, Second Edition.
Edited by Alan Glasper and Diane Carpenter.
© 2021 John Wiley & Sons Ltd. Published 2021 by John Wiley & Sons Ltd.
Companion website: www.wiley.com/go/glasper/nursingdissertation2e

Prudhoe, Cath Battrick and Edward Alan Glasper (2007). They have been encouraged to read it through first and then read it again more thoroughly to answer the questions posed by the appraisal tool.

Activity 18.1

Using your university library facilities go to the MAG online library Internurse collection site (https://www.magonlinelibrary.com/page/collections/internurse? utm_source=redirect&utm_medium=web&utm_campaign=internurse&) and source and print a copy of

Weaver, K., Prudhoe, G., Battrick, C. and Glasper, E.A. (2007) Sick children's perceptions of clown doctor humour. *British Journal of Nursing*, **1** (8), 359–365.

Most universities subscribe to Internurse and students can access papers free of charge. Additionally, this paper can be downloaded from the book student resource website.

Go to the CASP website and download and print a copy of the qualitative tool.

Screening questions

CASP tools always begin with two screening questions which, if they can be answered quickly with a 'Yes', suggest it is worth continuing with the full appraisal process. This is very helpful, as much time can be wasted on doing a full appraisal only to conclude that the article was not very rigorously written and little confidence may be had in its findings. If clinicians are thinking of changing their practice based on new evidence, they need to know that the research was sound. Greenhalgh (2019:6) warns of the dangers of clinical decision making by 'press cutting' and describes her experiences as a newly qualified doctor of keeping a file of papers from medical weeklies about new suggestions for clinical practice. She discusses how she would often change her practice based on what appeared to be the newest evidence but came to realise that she did not always know whether the studies to which the articles referred had been conducted rigorously or whether they were reliable.

With this in mind the students set about their task by looking at the screening questions. Sue looked at the first question, which asks whether there was a clear statement about the aims of the research. The CASP tool gives some hints to help answer this question: what was the research trying to discover, why was it important and to what extent was it relevant? Sue looked over the first few sentences of the clown article and thought she could see what it was aiming at. She then looked more closely at the abstract and found that the beginning of the second paragraph clearly stated that the focus of the study was 'the perceived effects of clown humour as experienced by children in a large children's inpatient facility in the South of England'. The main text gave her more specific details, that is, the study was part of a larger piece of work to investigate the impact of clown humour on children and their families and carers. It also provided some insights into why this study might be important and relevant. The authors had claimed that, firstly, there had been few studies to ascertain the therapeutic effects of using 'clown doctors' to relieve sick children's anxieties and, secondly, that there was little evidence to warrant the use of clown humour. She concluded she could answer 'Yes' to the first screening question.

The second screening question asks whether a qualitative methodology was appropriate. Greenhalgh's chapter on 'papers that go beyond numbers' (2019:165–178) gives a succinct overview about the relative merits of qualitative research and suggests that qualitative researchers 'seek a deeper truth' than that produced by exclusively quantitative research, which is interested in 'counting and measuring' perspectives. Qualitative researchers aim to study their participants in their natural setting (rather than in a contrived experimental situation) and are concerned with making sense of phenomena in terms of the meanings people attribute to them. They are keen to understand the complexities of human behaviour (Greenhalgh, 2019:165). Sam thought about this and noticed that the second paragraph of the article stated that crucial to the study 'was the idea of specifically seeking the views of the children themselves, on the benefits or otherwise of clown doctor humour' (p. 359). The study, then, was about children's experiences and data were collected from four wards (the children's 'natural' setting). Sam also concluded he could give an affirmative answer to the second screening question. Having shared their findings thus far, they concluded that the article had passed the screening process and they could progress to the eight detailed questions which followed.

The CASP qualitative questions

The first of these continued naturally from the question that Sam had considered so he agreed to answer it. It asked whether the study design was appropriate to address the aims of the research. The CASP tool suggests approaching this question by ascertaining whether the authors justified their research design. Did they, for instance, discuss how they chose their research method? Sam noted they had described the choice of 'draw and write/draw and tell' methods, which they stated were two complementary qualitative research designs. They gave a full account of the relative merits and criticisms of the approach with children, although they did not suggest any possible alternative study designs. However, the rationale for the choice of approach, Sam thought, had been given due and comprehensive consideration and was presented in a fair and non-biased way. Sam thus concluded that the research design was appropriate to address the aims of the research.

Meanwhile Charlotte was contemplating Question 4 of the CASP tool; this was the first of two questions addressing sampling and she had agreed to consider both. Question 4 focused on the recruitment strategy and whether it was appropriate to the aims of the research. To answer this question fully, Charlotte needed to discover whether the researchers had explained how the participants were selected and whether their recruitment had the potential to generate the type of knowledge sought by the study. The particular study the article referred to, although part of a larger research project which included experiences of parents and carers, was concerned with the child-patients' experiences of clown humour and whether it reduced their anxieties. Children were selected between the ages of four and eleven years, as this age group is suitable for engaging with the research methods of 'draw and write/ draw and tell'. Allowances were made for difficulties with writing and spelling. Eleven years was chosen as an upper age limit as it was thought that senior school children may have been exposed to more negative and 'horror' associations with clowns. The article also discussed the problems associated with recruitment. The researchers had approached 42 children but initially 16 did not consent to participate and a further six were unable to complete the second part of the data collection (they were discharged home early or felt too unwell). It was stated in the article that the data collection had been extended by a month to achieve just 20 participants. However, it was not clear to Charlotte why 20 children was the chosen number, although she guessed that this was all that were available to the team in the time frame allocated for the study. She had understood that in qualitative research participants were recruited until data saturation had been achieved. Charlotte did remind herself, however, that even though the article might not have given a complete account of why the number of participants had been selected, the authors were probably constrained by word limit. It was quite likely that the research itself gave due rationale. Had Charlotte been using the article for her evidence-based assignment then she would have contacted the researchers and asked them (contact details were provided in the article).

The fifth question, also concerned with sampling, included seven subsections. The overarching question addressing all of these subsections was whether the data were collected in a way that addressed the research issue. She had firstly to consider whether the setting for the data collection had been justified. Children had been selected from two medical and two surgical wards from a children's inpatient facility in the south of England. Further details were not to be gained from the article and Charlotte could not tell whether there were only four wards in this inpatient unit. Therefore, she did not think that the setting for the data had been entirely justified within the article. It was very clear, however, how the data were collected. This was the subject of the second subsection and Sue felt confident that the article had given a full description of how the 'draw and write/draw and tell' methods had been implemented and that data were collected about children's feelings on coming into hospital and, subsequently, following a visit from clown doctors (now known as giggle doctors because of the negative perceptions related to the word 'clown' in the media). The third subsection was concerned with justification of the methods chosen but this had already been addressed by Sam in Question 3. This puzzled Charlotte a little, but she concluded that the 'draw and write/draw and tell' approach was both a research design and a data collection method in a similar way to a survey. Charlotte thought the distinction between research design and data collection method in the article could have been a little clearer for the benefit of 'novice critical appraisers'. The fourth subsection asked whether the data collection methods were made explicit. Charlotte considered this had been demonstrated well in the article and illustrations had been provided for clarification. The fifth and sixth subsections addressed any modifications to the data collection methods during the study and whether the form of the data was clear. She could easily answer 'no' to the first and 'yes' to the second. The final area of 'sampling' for consideration was data saturation. This question had already been triggered for Charlotte under Question 4, so she felt she had already addressed this, although she stated here that there was no discussion in the article that data saturation had been achieved with 20 participants.

Reflexivity is the focus of Question 6 of the appraisal tool. Alisha had offered to consider this section and started with the first prompt, which was to determine whether the relationship between the researcher(s) and participants had been adequately considered. The principal data collector was a play therapist based at the hospital in which the study was conducted. The article made no reference to her having made a critical examination of her role, potential bias or influence, despite brief discussion in the methodology section of the difficulty for qualitative researchers not to impose their own views on the children who are the focus of the research. The article did make reference to the fact that the clown doctors (giggle doctors) were cognisant and supportive of the study, had no previous knowledge of which specific children were participating in the study and had no contact with the investigators. Thus, some potential for bias or influence was addressed but, importantly Alisha thought, not sufficiently focused on the play specialist's own potential for influence and interpretation. This section on reflexivity also requires consideration of how the researcher responded to events during the study and whether there were any changes in the research design. Other than

extending the period of study (already discussed) the article made no reference to this aspect. Alisha concluded that it is unlikely that any changes had
been made, as it would surely have been mentioned. She did agree with
Charlotte, however, that were she relying on this evidence to change practice
she would need to consult the primary data to be sure.

Ethical issues are addressed in Question 7 of the CASP checklist and
Alisha also considered the extent to which these had been taken into consideration. Some detail was given of how the research was explained to the children and that they were under no pressure to participate. Issues of consent
were also clearly addressed in the article but Alisha could find no evidence to
suggest that ethical permission had been sought from an appropriate NHS
ethics committee. The students had already discussed word constraints on
the authors but, notwithstanding this, decided this was an important omis-
sion on their part.

Data analysis

Data analysis was the next section and both Sue and Sam decided to tackle it
together. Question 8 (with six subsections) addressed this and asked whether
the analysis was sufficiently rigorous. The first three bullet-pointed hints
were straightforward to address: the article provided a reasonably in-depth
description of the process of analysis, a thematic analysis *was* used and Riley's
(1996) technique of coding data was used to delineate common themes. The
researchers described how the data presented were selected from the original
sample to demonstrate the analytical process. The fourth point asks whether
there was sufficient data presented to support the findings. Despite the article
being relatively short – just seven pages – Sue and Sam felt there was sufficient description to support the results. Two drawings by the same child were
also reproduced in the article to illustrate their findings. Both Sam and Sue
felt that here a picture painted a thousand words and that the reader could
immediately follow the authors' claims. Neither Sue nor Sam, however, considered that the authors had completely satisfied the next two parts of the
data analysis section. They both believed that there had been no discussion
of contradictory data and no critical examination of bias or influence in the
selection of data for presentation.

Research findings

Question 9 of the appraisal tool is concerned with the research findings and
asks whether there was a clear statement of these. Sue had searched the article for a specific section headed 'findings' but it eluded her, although she
deduced that this was contained in the discussion of results. On close reading

she considered the findings were clear and explicit and supported by two tables. Some discussion of the credibility of the findings was included but there appeared to be no discussion of the evidence for and against the researchers' arguments, although the findings were contextualised with respect to the original research questions. The authors claimed that 'the results of this qualitative study of clown humour show that sick children believe that it is generally positive in ameliorating their fears and apprehensions about their hospital admission'. Sue thought this rather a bold statement given that only 20 children had been studied and thought that their claims should have been modified to reflect the localised nature of the study.

The value of the research

The final section (Question 10) asks how valuable the research is and whether the researcher discussed the contribution the study makes to existing knowledge or understanding. All the students were clear that the authors had claimed that the study added to the growing literature base for the efficacy of clown humour as experienced by children in hospital. Sue also reminded the others that the limitations of the study were also identified and the authors had acknowledged that data were collected from children in only one hospital. Sam responded that this was not unusual in qualitative studies, which did not aim for their findings to be generalised. He stated that the question for those critiquing the article is to consider whether the findings are potentially transferable to their own clinical settings. To ascertain that they would have to consider the similarities in setting, geography, children's ages and other demographic variables for example. As the students were critically appraising the article as an exercise they were not able to draw any conclusions about this.

Reflection

When the students reflected on the process of critical appraisal they had undertaken they agreed that the research had some merits. They believed that the methodology was suitable for the nature of the enquiry and that the research had been conducted appropriately. The data collection was consistent with the methodological approach and addressed the research issue. They decided that the data analysis had also been conducted rigorously but that some important discussion points were missing from the article. One of the study's weakest areas appeared to be in the area of reflexivity. There seemed to have been little consideration of the relationship between researcher and participants and insufficient account made of the ethical considerations. On balance they concluded, as indeed the researchers had themselves, that further study was needed before any confidence could be given to the transferability of the findings or any change in practice made.

Having completed this exercise the students discussed how they might write up the process and outcomes of their critical appraisal. They had been advised that where they had several articles using the same research methodology they should initially complete individual appraisals on each of the articles, but when they wrote them up they should compare each article section by section. So, for instance, if they had five articles using a qualitative methodology, they should discuss all of them with respect to their satisfying the screening questions, and then the research design for each of them, and so on. They all felt more able to approach the task now and decided to make a start on appraising the qualitative articles they had found from their literature search and to structure their summaries according to the sections of the appraisal tool. Sue and Sam could see that this process would give them plenty of material for the 'discussion' section of their dissertations, as they would be able to comment on the relative strengths and weaknesses of each of the articles. This process would enable them to decide on balance whether there was enough 'good research' to support a change in practice. Alisha and Charlotte felt they had a better idea about how to discuss the relative strengths and weaknesses of research studies they cited in their assignments and were hopeful that this would help them to gain the higher grades they were keen to achieve.

References

CASP UK (2018a) Critical Appraisal Skills Programme, https://casp-uk.net/ (accessed 5 May 2020).

CASP UK (2018b) CASP Checklist: 10 questions to help you make sense of qualitative research. https://caspuk.net/wp-content/uploads/2018/01/CASP-Qualitative-Checklist-2018.pdf (accessed 5 May 2020).

Greenhalgh, T. (2019) *How to Read a Paper*, 6th edn. Blackwell Publishing, Oxford.

Riley, J. (1996) *Getting the Most from Your Data. A Handbook of Practical Ideas on How to Analyse Qualitative Data.* Technical and Educational Services Ltd.

Weaver, K., Prudhoe, G., Battrick, C. and Glasper, E.A. (2007) Sick children's perceptions of clown doctor humour. *British Journal of Nursing*, **1** (8), 359–365.

For further resources for this chapter visit the companion website at
www.wiley.com/go/glasper/nursingdissertation2e

Chapter 19 Critically reviewing quantitative papers using a CASP critiquing tool

Diane Carpenter[1] and Alan Glasper[2]

University of Plymouth, UK
University of Southampton, UK

Activity 19.1

From your university online library provision, source and print the journal paper:

Lattimer, V., George, S., Thompson, F. *et al.* (1998) General practice. Safety and effectiveness of nurse telephone consultation in out of hour's primary care: randomised controlled trial. *British Medical Journal*, **317**, 1054–1059.

Download from the CASP website (http://www.casp-uk.net/) a copy of the randomised controlled trial appraisal tool. (Chapter 18 gives more information on CASP.)

Use your highlighter pens to follow the narrative in this chapter.

Scenario

As part of a classroom activity all the students have been asked by their lecturers to critique an empirical paper using one of the CASP critiquing tools. The paper is based on a randomised controlled trial and Sue, Charlotte and Alisha are worried about the amount of numerical data within the paper. Sue is especially overawed by the questions posed within the critiquing tool and over coffee she and Sam confer. Sam has come across a *British Medical Journal* paper by Lattimer *et al.* (1998) and he uses this to help explain how to use the CASP critiquing tool.

This chapter is based on an earlier chapter by Steve George.

How to Write Your Nursing Dissertation, Second Edition.
Edited by Alan Glasper and Diane Carpenter.
© 2021 John Wiley & Sons Ltd. Published 2021 by John Wiley & Sons Ltd.
Companion website: www.wiley.com/go/glasper/nursingdissertation2e

SUE: 'Sam, this is really difficult. I don't even know what some of the questions mean, let alone the answers to them. Why does it have to be so complicated?'

SAM: 'It isn't complicated really Sue. What the CASP scheme does is to break down what is potentially a complex question into easily answerable bits. Come on, let's have a go'

Question 1   'Did the study ask a clearly focused question?'

SUE: 'Why is that important to ask as the first question? Aren't there more important things?'

SAM: 'No, the reason is that if the answer's 'No' you can stop reading at that point! If they haven't asked a clearly focused question they're not going to get an answer which means anything. So let's look at the question they've asked in this paper. Actually, they've phrased it as an objective. Their objective was:

To determine the safety and effectiveness of nurse telephone consultation in out of hours primary care by investigating adverse events and the management of calls.

SUE: 'Is that clearly focused enough?'

SAM: 'Well, what do you think?'

SUE: 'It sounds OK to me, but what do I know about it?'

SAM: 'It sounds OK to me too. If you look at what they've published previously they undertook a survey of general practitioner opinion a couple of years earlier, in which it became clear that the "safety" of putting nurses on the telephone to answer patients' calls was a concern amongst GPs at that time. It follows that a sensible aim of a large-scale study looking at nurse telephone consultation would be to establish its safety, and if they're going to do that it makes sense to do a study of effectiveness at the same time.'

SUE: 'I saw that they'd done the GP survey but then I noticed that they'd also done a pilot study previously. Why didn't they do the safety study at that stage?'

SAM: 'People often ask that. Generally speaking, when you're looking at the outcome of trials (NB: **clinical trials** are research studies performed with people and whose aim is to evaluate some kind of intervention, in this case nurse telephone consultation), the "effectiveness" outcomes are far more common than the "adverse event" outcomes by which we measure safety. In order to get to the adverse events we have to collect data on a large number of people – many more than would be included in a pilot study. Pilot studies are fine for establishing that the intervention will actually work (meaning that you can run it, not that it will be effective) and that the intervention will be acceptable, but not for establishing safety. In fact, many randomised controlled trials, even drug trials, don't look at safety – that's established much later by post-marketing surveillance studies. OK, you can rule out obvious toxicity early on in phase 1 and phase 2 trials, but not some of the rare side effects. You can look at effectiveness within a trial designed to measure safety, but not necessarily the other way around, because the numbers might not be enough.'

SUE: 'Hang on, hang on! Phase what?'

SAM: 'Sorry, getting a bit technical, but this is important stuff. Drug trials are classified into four types, generally speaking. Phase 1 trials are studies of small doses of new medicinal compounds in healthy volunteers and phase 2 trials are initial clinical studies in disease sufferers with the aim of establishing whether it's worth proceeding to a full-scale trial. Phase 3 trials, often incorporating analysis of things like cost-effectiveness of a new intervention, are the ones we generally think about as randomised controlled trials, and phase 4 trials aren't really trials at all: they're post-marketing surveillance studies designed to look at safety, usually of drugs, and including thousands of people.'

SUE: 'OK, so this is a phase 3 trial then?'

SAM: 'Yes, although safety was its primary outcome. The pharmaceutical terminology isn't used so often in non-drug intervention studies like this, and most non-drug trials are phase 3, although there's quite a case to be made for more early-phase studies of non-drug interventions. You might want to look at the Medical Research Council's guidance on developing and evaluating complex interventions, the last version of which came out in 2008. It's on their website.'

SUE: 'Right, I'll do that. What about the next question?'

Question 2 'Was this a randomised controlled trial and was it appropriately so?'

SUE: 'I get mixed up over this. You see, all of these people telephoned in, didn't they? They're not a random sample of the population at all.'

SAM: 'This is another one people often get wrong. Subjects in a randomised controlled trial *aren't* randomly selected from the population. There wouldn't be any point in doing that. If you were going to test a new antihypertensive drug you'd want all the subjects in your trial to have high blood pressure, and if you randomly selected them from the population they wouldn't. No, subjects in a randomised controlled trial are often highly selected, and "random", in this case, refers to the method by which you allocate them to treatment within the trial, not the means by which you select them from the population.'

SUE: 'Oh, I see. So "random" isn't about selection? That actually makes more sense. I'm looking at how they did the randomisation though, and it doesn't look like what I've seen before. Whenever I've looked at trials it seemed to be that patients were admitted to the trial, had their details taken, signed a consent form and were then given either one treatment or the other. But that's not what happened here is it?'

SAM: 'No, it isn't, but you've got to look at the way in which the intervention was set up and consider the alternatives. In order to do what you've just described the investigators would have had to set up two services, one using nurses on the telephone, one not, working in parallel, at the same time, and sent each patient to one of them or the other. That would have been very costly to do, if not logistically impossible. So they did what was possible and split the year up into periods when the nurse telephone service was available and periods when it wasn't .'

SUE: 'But is that random? How did they randomise?'

SAM: 'They used a method called "block randomisation". This is often done in drug trials in order to iron out differences in numbers of subjects in each arm of a trial (arm 1 the intervention, i.e. the nurse-led telephone service, and arm 2 the regular doctor-led telephone service). Rather than using a completely random sequence of numbers the trial is divided into blocks of four or six subjects, commonly, and within each block two (of four) or three (of six) subjects are allocated to each intervention. Allocation within each block is random, so the whole sequence of all the blocks placed one after another becomes random.'

SUE: 'But why not just use a random sequence of numbers?'

SAM: 'Because it can result in quite considerable differences of numbers in differ-ent arms of trials, particularly if a trial is small. I remember well a student pilot trial in which they only intended to recruit 20 patients. The trouble is, they used a simple random sequence and ended up with 19 people in one arm and only one in the other. Essentially it meant that the study was use-less! That can't happen with block randomisation'

SUE: 'That sounds like a good idea then. But does block randomisation ever lead to problems?'

SAM: 'It can do, in that if it is known that a trial is block randomised in, say, blocks of four, it becomes possible to predict to which group the last case in a block is allocated. A clinician wishing to push a patient into one treatment group or another might therefore be able to move patients around to get their chosen patient into their preferred group. You get around that by using a mixture of blocks of different sizes, say four and six, so it becomes impos-sible to predict.'

SUE: 'And how did they do it in this study?'

SAM: 'They used a method I'd not seen before – in fact, it might have been the first time it had been used. They divided the year over which they were going to run the trial into a series of 26 blocks of two weeks. Within each block they therefore had two Monday evenings, two Tuesday evenings, two weekends, and so on. They then randomised so that one or other of the two became a period during which the service ran. Each one of those evenings or weekends became an allocation unit within the trial, with the patients ringing in during that block allocated to one service or the other. They obtained consent on behalf of the patients from the participating general practitioners.'

SUE: 'So this is a phase 3 block randomised controlled trial? How do I tell whether or not the randomisation was appropriate?'

SAM: 'There are two questions here – firstly, was a randomised trial the appropri-ate way of answering this question and, secondly, was the way in which it was done appropriate? You'll have seen the Cochrane Hierarchy of Evidence in which the *quality of the evidence* is determined by the methods used to minimise bias within a study design?'

SUE: 'Yes, and it puts the randomised controlled trial nearly at the top of the evidence tree. They call it the "gold standard" for research.'

SAM: 'Yes, that's right, but it's the gold standard only for the question "*How effective (or safe) is a new treatment in the management of a specified ailment compared to a placebo or to the best existing treatment?*" For other questions other research designs are better. A randomised controlled trial won't answer the question "What is the cause of this rare disease?" and it won't tell you why patients don't like, say, turning up to antenatal clinics. The first of those questions is best addressed by a case–control study and the second by, most likely, a qualitative study in the first instance, possibly followed up by a survey designed using data from the qualitative study. Even in the case of effectiveness of an intervention a single randomised controlled trial is bettered by a systematic review of several well-designed randomised controlled trials. However, in this case, a randomised controlled trial was the best way to answer the question set, and there hadn't been a previous trial on this subject with which it could be included in a systematic review.'

SUE: 'Fine, I understand that now. And did they do it appropriately?'

Question 3 'Were participants appropriately allocated to intervention and control groups?'

SAM: 'Well, you can look at what they did, but the best way to tell if randomisation has been effective is to look at the tables of baseline data for a trial – often Table 1, but in this paper split between Tables 2 and 3. As a broad rule, if the two groups randomised are broadly similar randomisation has worked, and if they're not, it hasn't.'

SUE: 'It looks as if it worked in this case then.'

SAM: 'I would say so. The numbers in each group overall are similar and there are only a few minor differences between numbers in different age groups, which I doubt influenced results in any important fashion. If there *had* been differences it would have been important to look at how participants were allocated to the intervention and control groups, whether the process was truly random, whether the method of allocation was described, whether any method was used to balance the randomization, like stratification, how the randomization schedule was generated and how a participant was allocated to a study group. Now, what about blinding?'

Question 4 'Were participants, staff and study personnel "blind" to participants study group?'

SUE: 'I find blinding a difficult subject. Perhaps I'm just stupid.'

SAM: 'Nonsense – the reason you find it difficult is that it *is* difficult, more so than some people realise. When you're assessing blinding you not only have to think about whether blinding was absent or present but also who was blinded and who wasn't, and what the potential effect of non-blinding would be in each case. And people also fail to separate "blinding" from "allocation concealment", which can have different effects on a trial. You also have to consider, if you're ever going to conduct a trial, what you can do to minimise the effects of non-blinding.'

SUE: 'Go on, remind me about blinding. . .'

SAM: 'OK. Quick explanation coming up! A blinded trial is one in which the design prevents participants, carers or those assessing outcome from knowing which intervention group a participant was in. Blinding is sometimes impossible, for instance in trials of surgical operations – ethically, "sham procedures", in which a patient ends up with the external signs of having had an operation in the form of a scar but where no procedure was performed, are definitely frowned upon. Also, trials of therapies involving active patient participation, like "talking therapies" or physiotherapy, can't be blinded easily.'

SUE: 'And what about "single blind" and "double blind" trials?'

SAM: 'I'm glad you asked that, but it's really historical now. Various studies reported that different authors used those terms – and also used "triple blind" – but meant different things by the terms. For instance, some authors used "single blind" to mean that subjects in the trial were blinded to what they were getting but those running the trial or assessing the outcome weren't, but others used it to mean exactly the opposite. The 2010 CONSORT (CONsolidated Standards of Reporting Trials) Statement recommended that the use of these terms be terminated and that reports of trials which were meant to be blinded should discuss instead "If done, who was blinded after assignment to interventions (for example, participants, care providers, those assessing outcomes) and how?" '

SUE: 'And what about the effects of non-blinding?'

SAM: 'Well the main effect of non-blinding is primarily on assessment of outcomes, and so the magnitude of the effect depends on how subjective, or not, an outcome is. A patient in a trial of an agent designed to help them stop smoking might be more inclined to report that they've stopped if they know they've had the active intervention. Likewise, a researcher assessing a patient and who knew they'd been on the active intervention might be more inclined to report a favourable outcome because they have a vested interest in finding one. However, if you have a blood test to tell you whether or not they've been smoking that is much less subjective and so non-blinding doesn't matter so much.'

SUE: 'I can't see how they might have blinded this trial.'

SAM: 'No, and they don't claim to have blinded it. It's pretty obvious whether or not you spoke straightaway to a doctor or whether or not you spoke to a nurse first, or only to a nurse. But the outcomes were all pretty much objective, total deaths, got from death certificates, and numbers of A&E attendances and hospital admissions, so it's unlikely to matter that it wasn't blinded. But while we're on the subject let's talk about "allocation concealment", which is the procedure for protecting the randomisation process so that the treatment to be allocated is not known before a patient is entered into the study. In this case the pattern of intervention was known only to the lead investigators throughout the study. Nurses and doctors working within the GP practice on the ground were blind to the intervention until a point when they would be unable to choose or swap duty periods, so, for instance, a doctor couldn't decide that they weren't going to work on a night when the nurse service was working, or not. The doctor or nurse pattern was not publicised anywhere and only became apparent to members of the public on the day of calling.'

SUE: So is that enough?'

SAM: 'In the context of this trial I think it's the best that could be done. Right, onwards and upwards! Next question.'

Question 5   'Were all the participants who entered the trial accounted for at its conclusion?'

SUE: 'Doesn't that always happen?'

SAM: 'No, it doesn't, unfortunately. It's always worth checking. Have you heard of intention-to-treat (ITT) analysis?'

SUE: 'Vaguely. . .'

SAM: 'Mmm. Well, ITT analysis means that all the patients who were enrolled and randomly allocated to the intervention were included in the analysis and were analysed in the groups to which they were randomised. But people vary in the way in which they interpret the term. In order to do ITT analysis properly you need to account for *every* person who was recruited to the trial and make sure they were analysed in the group to which they were first assigned, not the one in which they ended up – which in drug trials can be different for various reasons – and that they're not left out because, for instance, they didn't complete the course of treatment. In this trial people were entered according to the system in operation at the time they called, so swapping groups isn't really an option, and all the tables add up, so nobody in this trial was left out of the analysis. Next question. . .'

Chapter 19

Question 6   'Were the participants in all groups followed up and data collected in the same way?'

SUE: 'I've looked at this and I can't see that they were treated differently in any way.'

SAM: 'I would say that they were treated the same way. The investigators seem to have collected data on workload from the database of calls, data on mortality from the Office for National Statistics, data on admissions from local hospitals and then data on attendance at A&E from the GP cooperative records, all using the total list of names and addresses of people that had called, and they then matched the data gathered to the period in which they called, so it would have been difficult to treat them differently.'

SUE: 'And how about Question 7?'

Question 7   'Did the study have enough participants to minimise the play of chance?'

SAM: 'Well from your point of view the first thing to look out for is that they've done a sample size calculation before starting the trial. Then, look to see if they actually achieved that sample size during recruitment. In this trial they did both, so I'd give that box a tick. Statisticians use specialist software to calculate sample sizes and unless it's something quite simple you're unlikely to be able to replicate the calculation by yourself. So, unless you're planning on becoming a statistician and spending quite a lot of money on software, I'd leave it at that! Question 8 then. . .'

Question 8 'How are the results presented and what is the main result?'

SAM: 'OK. What did they find?'

SUE: 'I found this difficult as well, because they say this is an equivalence trial, and I'd never heard of one of those'.

SAM: 'Yes, equivalence trials are a subject area all to themselves. But they're not that hard once you know the basics. The first part to get around is that you can't prove that two treatments have exactly the same effect.'

SUE: 'Why not?'

SAM: 'Because in order to do that you'd need an infinite number of people in each arm of the trial. And that's not just one infinite number of people, that's two infinite numbers of people!'

SUE: 'Oh, so what do you do then?'

SAM: 'You have to specify a range within which you believe that a difference in clinical effect is of no importance. There are various ways of doing that, which seem to range from just pulling a number out of a hat to looking at patient estimates of whether an effect is important. That's particularly useful when you're looking at patient-reported outcomes. A lot depends on being able to specify the "minimal important clinical difference". This can be done using information gathered from previous papers, or from pilot studies.'

SUE: 'And what about this paper?'

SAM: 'They looked at the existing death rate for England and calculated an expected number of deaths based on the size of the population covered by the GP cooperative used for the trial – that in itself is quite a small number of deaths. They then set limits around it from 80 to 125% of that number, which is a range used in bioequivalence studies.'

SUE: 'So to show equivalence they just had to show a number of deaths between those limits?'

SAM: 'Not quite – they had to show a number of deaths *plus the confidence intervals around it* between the equivalence limits. And those confidence intervals are the key to understanding equivalence trials, and why they tend to be much bigger than trials designed to show a difference.'

SUE: 'Go on. . .'

SAM: 'You see, everybody wants to specify the narrowest pair of equivalence limits they can, but in order to do that you need to get a very narrow confidence interval around whatever you're measuring as the outcome of the trial, and trying to achieve a narrower confidence always means getting more people into the study.'

SUE: 'I see. And they did show equivalence I see. What would have happened if they hadn't? Would they have been able to say that the two interventions were different?'

SAM: 'Not necessarily. They might have, but only if the area covered by the confidence intervals lay completely outside the area defined by the equivalence limits. If the confidence intervals crossed either equivalence limit they'd have had to have said that they were uncertain whether there was equivalence or not.'

SUE: 'And that would mean that there was no statistically significant difference?'

SAM: 'Again, not necessarily. They could have a statistically significant difference, because the confidence intervals did not include the line of no difference. But if it crossed one of the equivalence limits, the difference, although significant, might not be important. And statistical significance and clinical importance aren't the same thing.'

SUE: 'But when you see difference trials reported they usually just tell you about the significant result they've got.'

SAM: 'Quite true. In that way equivalence trials are more honest than difference trials, because you have to state at the outset when you're planning your trial and what you consider to be important differences, whereas, as you say, difference trials often don't tell you at all whether they think the difference they've found is important.'

SUE: 'And is that what they did for all the outcomes?'

SAM: 'Yes, they did, with equivalence limits and confidence intervals, and confidence intervals bring us onto the next question.'

Question 9 'How precise are these results?'

SUE: 'Haven't we just done that?'

sam: 'We have, but in a difference trial we might by now have looked at the magnitude of the result but not at the confidence intervals around it.'

SUE: 'And can we make a decision using the results we've seen?'

SAM: 'Well I think we ought to move on to the final question before answering that. . .'

Question 10 'Were all important outcomes considered so the results can be applied?'

SUE: 'I think that they did consider all the important outcomes. Let's see, they looked at deaths within seven days of a contact with the out-of-hours service, emergency hospital admissions within 24 hours and within three days of contact, attendance at A&E within three days of a contact and how all the calls were managed and by whom. Isn't that enough?'

SAM: 'Yes, I think it is. But what you've got to ask is "What decision am I being asked to make?" This trial was the first one to look at the safety of nurse telephone consultation services. However, the results have to be looked at in light of the service being tested. In this trial the nurses worked within the context of a primary care cooperative, and they haven't existed since the change in GP contracts a few years ago removed GPs' responsibility for out-of-hours care. So, the result showing that calls needing to be handled by doctors were reduced by 50% can't now be interpreted, unless a similar system comes into operation again. One of the major problems with randomised controlled trials is that their results are too often applied to people who weren't represented in the trial population, or in circumstances which are different from those pertaining in the trial.'

SUE: 'Oh. So is there nothing we can learn from this trial any more?'

SAM: 'I'm not saying that. The major concern prior to the trial was about the safety of nurses undertaking telephone consultation and that result still stands. But the results of this trial were used by the government to inform the setting up of the now disbanded NHS Direct, which wasn't linked to primary care and consequently never showed the reduction in workload for out-of-hours medical care.'

SUE: 'OK. That's an important lesson. Thanks Sam.'

All the students found the CASP tool to be helpful in understanding the mechanisms of randomised controlled trials.

For further resources for this chapter visit the companion website at
     www.wiley.com/go/glasper/nursingdissertation2e

Chapter 20 **Critically reviewing a journal paper using the Parahoo model**

Diane Carpenter[1] and Alan Glasper[2]
[1]*University of Plymouth, UK*
[2]*University of Southampton, UK*

> **Scenario**
> The students are investigating which critiquing tool to use for the analysis of their selected scholarly papers. Sam has read some of the work of Professor Kader Parahoo, who is Research Director at the Institute of Nursing and Health Research at the University of Ulster. They are interested in using his model of critiquing, which is discussed in more detail in this chapter.

Introduction

Evidence-based practice depends, amongst other things, on researchers providing robust evidence from their studies. To decide whether a study has been rigorously carried out and whether its findings are relevant for your practice, you need to develop critical appraisal skills. The terms 'appraisal' or 'evaluation' of a published research paper are often used interchangeably to refer to the process of judging the quality of a study and its relevance for one's practice.

This chapter is based on an earlier chapter by Kader Parahoo and Irene Heuter.

How to Write Your Nursing Dissertation, Second Edition.
Edited by Alan Glasper and Diane Carpenter.
© 2021 John Wiley & Sons Ltd. Published 2021 by John Wiley & Sons Ltd.
Companion website: www.wiley.com/go/glasper/nursingdissertation2e

Scenario

The students also undertake this activity and Sam finds an exemplar of the critiquing exercise with which to assess their own endeavours.

Framework for appraisal

There are many tools for appraising or evaluating research studies (e.g. CASP, 2018; ScHARR, 2018; SIGN, 2019). In this chapter, the framework provided by Parahoo (2006, chapter 17, Evaluating research studies) will be used to appraise the Rice *et al.* (2008) paper. The framework consists of a number of headings (listed below), which are based on the structure that is most often used to report both qualitative and quantitative studies in research journals and as such can be considered as a generic critiquing tool for most research articles.

- Title of study
- Abstract
- Literature review/Background
- Methodology or Design
- Results
- Discussion and interpretation (including limitations)
- Recommendations

Title of study

Does the title convey the study clearly and accurately?
The title of this paper reflects a study that tests the effects of a preoperative education programme (independent variable) on preoperative anxiety (dependent variable) in children (the population). Therefore, the title contains all the key components in this study (the variables, the type of relationship

between them, i.e. 'effect', and the population). The title also identifies the design of the study (observational).

From the title can I decide whether this paper is relevant to my practice?
If I work in paediatric care where induction of anaesthesia is carried out, then this study is highly relevant to me.

Abstract

Does the abstract give a short and concise summary of the following aspects of the study?
- *Background.* The study is put in context by pointing out the distress and potential harm to children who have to receive anaesthesia. Some of the strategies used to minimise anxiety in children are mentioned and the authors briefly state that a Saturday Morning Club (SMC) has been in existence at their own hospital to address this issue.
- *Aim.* The aim was 'to assess the influence of attendance at a Saturday Morning Club (the preoperative education programme) on anxiety in patients aged between 2 and 16 years'.
- *Designs.* An observational study design was used. Patient anxiety was measured by the modified Preoperative Anxiety Scale; parental anxiety was self-reported and assessed by means of a visual analogue scale. The assessment time points were on the day ward, in the preoperative waiting room and at induction of anaesthesia. The sample comprised 94 children aged between 2 and 16 years old. Twenty-one attended the SMC and 73 did not. We are told that observers were unaware (blinded) of who had attended or not. There is also mention of the statistical test: the Mann–Whitney U-test.
- *Results.* The results are briefly and clearly presented. Attendance was reported as having had a 'favourable effect' on patient anxiety, but that this was only statistically significant in the waiting room. However, the results for parental anxiety were not given in the abstract.
- *Conclusions.* Further studies are recommended to provide evidence to support the use of a preoperative education programme. However, the authors do not comment on the evidence produced by this study.

Overall the abstract is well written and presented. It is a very good example of how an abstract can be short and yet provide readers with relevant information for them to decide whether the study has some merit and is worth reading.

Chapter 20

Scenario

Alisha was wondering whether it would be possible to write her final assignment by just looking at the abstracts of journal articles as they provide such useful summaries. Charlotte said that her lecturer had addressed this and strongly advised against it as it is still possible to have a well-written abstract, but on closer evaluation of the whole article to discover that the research was not conducted rigorously. Sue agreed and reminded them that clinical decisions should be based on evidence and it is the responsibility of trained health professionals to ensure that any advice they give or changes to practice they consider are based on the best quality of evidence.

Literature review/Background

Is the importance of study justified?
The authors justify the importance of this study by identifying (in the first four sentences of the introduction) the main stress-related problems associated with the induction of anaesthesia in children. Relevant studies are appropriately referenced. Some of the listed problems included are physiological, physical and psychological. The authors mention nightmares, eating disorders, enuresis and behavioural problems. The link between parental anxiety and children's distress is also briefly mentioned.

What is the context of this study?
This study was carried out to investigate the effect of an existing preoperative educational programme (in the form of an SMC) on children about to undergo day-case surgery. The programme is itself briefly described. The information given is adequate for readers to understand what the programme entails.

Does the literature review show the gap(s) in knowledge which this study seeks to fill?
With reference to the literature, the authors list the main strategies used to reduce anxiety. These include premedication, parental presence at induction, psychological preparation and preoperative education (leaflets, books or play therapy). There is no indication of whether all or any of these have an effect on children's anxiety. However, in the discussion section, we are informed that 'several studies have demonstrated the efficacy of premedication' (p. 428). The authors state in the discussion that 'preoperative education programmes are costly' and that 'evidence of their benefit is variable' (p. 428). It would have been helpful if this information was provided in the introduction.

Presumably the SMC is the first of its kind (but we are not told this in the introduction).

Aims/objectives/research questions/hypotheses

Are the aims of the study clear?
The main aim of the study is clear (see the last sentence under Introduction). The study investigated the effect of the education programme on anxiety in children undergoing day-care surgery. There is, however, no mention of the other aim, which is to measure parental anxiety as well. At this stage it is not clear if the authors intend to assess the relationship between children's distress and parental anxiety.

Scenario

Charlotte and Alisha check their understanding with Sam and Sue. They were a little confused because they thought that the Parahoo framework could be used as a generic appraisal tool, but they know that qualitative research studies do not have hypotheses. Sam reassured them that they would delete as appropriate from this section and that they could expect a qualitative study to have a question (although sometimes only a topic is referred to) as well as aims and objectives.

Chapter 20

Design of study

What is the design of the study? Is it the most appropriate for the aims of the study?
A prospective observational study design was selected. The National Institutes of Health (2017) defines an observational study as:

> *a study in which the investigators do not intervene, but simply observe the course of events over time. That is, investigators do not manipulate the use of, or deliver, an intervention or exposure (e.g., do not assign patients to treatment and control groups), but only observe patients who [receive] (and sometimes patients who [do] not, as a basis of comparison) . . . the intervention or exposure, and interpret the outcomes. These studies are more subject to selection bias than experimental studies such as randomized controlled trials.*

This type of design is appropriate for evaluating the effects of an intervention or practice which was already in place. Under 'Limitations of study', the authors explain that it was thought 'to be unethical to conduct an RCT' as the SMC was 'an established facility' in the hospital.

This study is prospective because the participants were 'followed' from the time they attended the SMC (two weeks before surgery) to the time they came for elective surgery.

The strength of an observational study is that researchers do not seek to manipulate the situation (i.e. change normal practice to carry out the experiment). Instead, in observational studies, researchers study real-life situations.

In an observational study, researchers do not have control over the selection and allocation of participants to groups. For example, in this case an SMC was already offered to parents and children who decided to attend or not. Observational studies are therefore prone to selection bias. For this reason the evidence from observational studies is not considered to be as strong as that from good randomised controlled trials (RCTs).

However, observational studies can 'indicate' whether an intervention works and this can be further tested by RCTs (as recommended by the authors of this study).

Are the main concepts (to be measured) defined?

The main concept measured is the 'distress' (DAI) of children. No operational definition of 'distress' is given but an anxiety scale is used to measure distress. One could ask if 'distress' and 'anxiety' can be used interchangeably.

What are the methods of data collection? Are they constructed for the purpose of the current study or do the researchers use existing ones?

The main instrument used in this study was the 'modified Yale Preoperative Anxiety Scale' (mYPAS) to measure anxiety in children preoperatively and at induction of anaesthesia. Parental anxiety was self-reported using a 100-mm visual analogue scale (VAS).

The use of the Yale Preoperative Anxiety Scale (YPAS) was justified because 'it is sensitive to changes in anxiety over time' and it has 'good inter-observer reliability and high construct concurrent validity' (p. 427). What is not clear, however, is who modified the YPAS. Was it the researchers in this study? Or was there a modified version? If the latter, there is no reference for it. If the former, why was it modified and how does this affect the internal consistency of the original YPAS?

The justification for the use of the VAS for measuring parental anxiety was because it 'is widely used and has good validity when compared with other assessment methods' (p. 429).

Who collected data? Can this introduce bias in the study?

To avoid observation bias, two observers who were blinded to the study were used (i.e. they did not know who participated in the SMC or not).

To minimise observation errors and achieve a degree of consistency between the two observers, a pilot study was performed to assess inter-observer reliability. The Kappa test 'showed excellent agreement between the two observers' scores' (p. 427).

In studies where there is more than one group, is there a description of what intervention/treatment each group receives?
In this study, both groups (SMC attenders and non-attenders) received the same care and treatment, although the anaesthetist and anaesthetic management were not standardised. In a study of real-life situations (as in this case) it is neither practical nor ethical to interfere with the care and treatment which the health service provides for patients.

The data collected for the two groups (demographic details, use of sedatives, etc.) were well described.

Is the setting(s) where the study is carried out adequately described?
The setting, procedures and policies are all adequately described. This information helps the reader to understand the context of the study and to compare with their own settings (in case they want to introduce the SMC at their own hospital).

Who was selected? From what population were they selected? What was the precise method of selection and allocation? Was there a sample size calculation?
As explained earlier, in observational studies researchers have little control over the selection and allocation of participants to groups. In this study participants were recruited on the day of surgery. Every child who came for treatment was observed (whether they participated previously in the SMC or not). Only those 'who did not speak English as a first language and those who had severe developmental delay' (p. 427) were excluded. There is no information about the target population. For example, while we are told that only 25% of families chose to attend the SMC, there is no indication of how many families attended the SMC monthly or annually.

Their rationale for the sample size (*n* = 94) is not given, although (in 'Limitations') the authors express the view that it was 'not possible to state with any degree of certainty what reduction in the mYPAS scores would be clinically significant' and that was the reason why 'a power analysis was not undertaken' (p. 429). In addition, it is not noted which mYPAS score range is considered to represent 'moderate' or 'severe' anxiety. Such a classification could have been employed in a sample size estimation.

Was ethical approval obtained? Are there any other ethical implications?
Ethical approval was obtained from the institutional ethics committee. Informed consent was obtained from parents and children. As there is no mention of refusal from any parent or child, we can only assume that they all agreed to participate.

Those whose first language was not English and those with 'severe developmental delay' were excluded. It is possible that these two groups may have greater anxiety because of communication problems. Their needs should also be taken into account through research.

Scenario

Sam told the others that quite often research articles do not mention whether ethical approval was sought and granted. Often this is because of word limitations imposed by journal publishers and if reviewers are in any doubt they should contact the article's authors.

Data analysis

Was there a separate section in the paper that explained the planned analyses prior to the presentation of the results?
We are only told in the results section which statistical methods were used and how they were applied to the data. Most of this information can be gathered in the four separate tables that summarise (i) patient demographic data, (ii) patient baseline characteristics, (iii) patients anxiety scores by attenders/non-attenders and (iv) parental anxiety VAS scores by attenders/non-attenders.

Which statistical methods were relied on?
Generally, continuous variables, such as age, patient anxiety scores and parental anxiety VAS scores, were summarised by the median and interquartile range. The Mann–Whitney U-test was used to compare these variables between the two groups of SMC attenders and non-attenders. Categorical variables, such as number of male patients and number of patients who previously had general anaesthesia, were summarised by frequency counts and percentages. The Fisher exact test was used to compare categorical variables between the two groups of SMC attenders and non-attenders. P-values are determined to be statistically significant if they do not exceed 0.05.

It is suitable to list the median and interquartile range as summary statistics for the variables that are analysed via the Mann–Whitney U-test, because this is a non-parametric test and compares the difference in the medians of the two groups. The column header of Table 1 that says 'Kruskal Wallis test' is a bit confusing. Firstly, since there are two groups, the header should have stated 'Mann–Whitney U-test'. Secondly, it is not clear how the Kruskal-Wallis test could have been applied to the categorical variables 'Total number of SMC attenders' and 'Number of male patients'.

Is it clear how the statistical tests were applied to the data and groups?
The table presentation clearly identifies the variables, groups, statistical tests performed and the resulting test results (here, P-values). It is easy for the reader to follow.

Scenario

Charlotte asked how they would answer this question for a qualitative study. Sam, who is very keen on qualitative research, suggested she look up data analysis for qualitative studies and refer to that. He said that often the data were analysed thematically, but that there were different approaches to this. He said it was always useful to have a research methods textbook to hand when critically appraising.

Results

Are the results clearly presented?
The results in the text and in the tables are clearly presented.

As usual for this type of study, the demographic details and other parameters, such as previous history of general anaesthesia, method of anaesthesia, parental presence at induction, use of premedication and so on, are provided. This allows readers to assess whether the two groups were similar in these respects.

Are the results for all the aims presented?
The aims were to measure patient and parent anxiety. The results of both these aims are provided.

Are the results fully presented?
In addition to the results stated about the statistical significance of the group comparisons at each time point, one could have mentioned a noticeable increasing trend in the anxiety levels in the SMC non-attenders group for both patients and parents, which is much less emphasised in the SMC attenders group. For example, the medians stay the same (or nearly the same) in the waiting area as in the day ward for the SMC attenders, while the same medians markedly increase for the SMC non-attenders.

Scenario

Alisha said that she supposed the same principle was true for the results section as with the analysis. Sue replied that often quotes extracted from interviews would be presented to demonstrate the themes following analyses. Quantitative results are typically presented in tables whereas qualitative results are usually in a narrative format.

Chapter 20

Discussion

Most of the statements in the 'Discussion' section are about the variety of methods to address anxiety associated with anaesthesia and their effectiveness. Most of this should have been in the Introduction/Background. The 'real' discussion in this study is under the heading 'Limitations'.

Is it a balanced discussion? Have all possible explanations for the results been given?

Overall, it is a well-balanced discussion. The authors offer a number of ways to interpret the results. However, they do not elaborate as to why they think a type II error could account for the failure to detect a statistically significant difference between the score of the two groups on the day ward and in the anaesthetic room.

Are the results discussed in the context of previous studies?

The design and findings of a number of relevant studies are discussed in an attempt to put the findings of this study in the context of what is already known on this topic. Readers are therefore provided with information on other similar studies to follow up, if they wish.

Are the results fully discussed?

While the authors mention that the 'present study has shown that children who have attended our preadmission education programme (the SMC) have statistically significant lower anxiety levels in the waiting area than those who have not attended the SMC', this finding has not been leveraged against the findings that SMC non-attenders generally were older and had previously had anaesthesia. This could have impacted the results based on statistical inference in either way if these factors were incorporated in the analysis. We do not know.

It is mentioned in the 'Limitations' later on that possibly the older children in this study, who are also more likely to have received a previous general anaesthetic, have already attended the SMC. This remains speculation, since unfortunately the number of patients who previously attended the SMC and the number of patients who previously had general anaesthesia were not recorded in this study. This is somewhat of a shortcoming of this study and should be built into any future (randomised) trial.

Are the limitations of the study discussed?

The authors point out that it was not possible to conduct an RCT and give reasons for this. They also admit that no data were recorded on whether some of the older children had received a previous general anaesthetic or may have attended the SMC on an earlier occasion.

Another limitation which the authors identify is that they did not take into account the relationship between the timing of the programme (SMC) and the age of children, as younger children may have shorter recall times.

Conclusions/Recommendations

Are the conclusions justified?
The authors are justified in claiming that the results show their programme (attendance at the SMC) reduced patient anxiety in the waiting area. The design of the study is robust enough for readers to reach this conclusion.

Are there recommendations for policy, practice or further research?
The authors recommend a larger RCT to examine the cost-effectiveness of this programme in the UK setting. They could also have recommended that future studies include those whose primary language is not English and also other vulnerable groups, such as children with physical and/or mental disability, where possible.

Are the results/conclusions helpful for my practice?
In the absence of more robust evidence, the findings of this study (less anxiety among those who attended the SMC, especially in the waiting area) could be used to inform practice. Evidence-based practice takes into account (Sackett *et al.*, 1996):

- evidence from research;
- clinical expertise;
- patients' preferences and wishes.

Any decision to implement the findings should also take into account the cost of the SMC. Although all these factors are important, the findings of this study should increase confidence when contemplating the possibility of implementing such a programme.

Are the results generalisable?
The results are not generalisable to all children, since those who attended the SMC were self-selective. Only 25% of those offered the SMC attended. Among these, it is not clear which age group benefited the most. In this study the ages of children ranged from 2 to 16. Being at different developmental stages, it is unlikely that such programmes affect these children in the same way. Further analysis of the data and future research could shed more light on the effects of such programmes on younger and older children.

Chapter 20

> ### Scenario
>
> The students also discussed this point because they knew that the study they had been asked to look at was quantitative, but that qualitative research does not aim to be generalisable. This is mainly because the sample sizes are typically too small and the data are analysed differently so that statistical significance cannot be determined. Instead, they agreed, in appraising a qualitative study, they would ask to what extent the findings were transferable. This, they understood, meant that they should ask whether the profile of the participants and the clinical context were similar to the clinical areas they were working in. Sam raised the point that it would be unusual to change practice based on the results of a qualitative study. Instead, it might indicate where further studies needed to be conducted.

Funding

Is there potential conflict of interest (if information on funding is provided)?
No information on who funded this study is provided.

Conclusion

This study seemed to have served its purpose by providing information on whether anxiety at induction was influenced by attendance at an SMC two weeks previously. In some ways one could describe it as a pilot study (e.g. the sample was quite small) which raised a number of questions that could be more rigorously investigated by a large RCT. Nonetheless, the quality of this study itself is good enough for the findings to be taken seriously.

References

Critical Appraisal Skills Programme (CASP) (2018) CASP Appraisal Checklists. https://casp-uk.net/casp-tools-checklists/ (accessed 27 February 2020).

National Institutes of Health (2017) National Information Center on Health Services Research and Health Care Technology (NICHSR) Glossary. http//www.nlm.nih.gov/nichsr/hta101/ta101014.html (accessed 27 February 2020).

Parahoo, K. (2006) *Nursing Research: Principles, Process and Issues*, 2nd edn. Palgrave, Basingstoke, UK.

Rice, M., Glasper, A., Keeton, D. and Spargo, P. (2008) The effect of a preoperative education programme on perioperative anxiety in children: an observational study. Pediatric Anesthesia, **18**, 426–430.

Sackett, D.L., Rosenberg, W.M.C., Muir Gray, J.A. *et al.* (1996) Evidence based medicine: what it is and what it isn't. British Medical Journal, **312**, 71–72.

School of Health and Related Research (ScHARR) (2018), http://www.shef.ac.uk/scharr/ (accessed 27 February 2020).

Scottish Intercollegiate Guidelines Network (SIGN) (2019), https://www.sign.ac.uk/what-we-do/methodology/checklists/ (accessed on 27 February 2020).

For further resources for this chapter visit the companion website at
www.wiley.com/go/glasper/nursingdissertation2e

Chapter 20

Section 6   **Taking your dissertation further: disseminating evidence, knowledge transfer; writing as a professional skill**

Just when Charlotte and Alisha thought they had completed the difficult parts of their assignments, they realised they still had to write a reflective element. They agreed it is easy to overlook the smaller compnents of the set work and to leave themselves little time for it. They have come to realise the importance of reflection and Charlotte discusses frameworks that might help get them started. Sue and Sam have a similar conversation and help each other to apply Gibbs' cycle of reflection to their work.

Chapter 21 Publishing your work or making a conference or poster presentation

Diane Carpenter[1] and Alan Glasper[2]
[1]*University of Plymouth, UK*
[2]*University of Southampton, UK*

Scenario

The students are really pleased that they have completed their courses and their dissertations and final projects/assignments. They had all worked hard and this represented a real achievement for them. Sam did especially well and achieved a high grade for his dissertation and his supervisor has suggested that he should consider thinking about presenting at a local conference and perhaps send a paper for peer review to a nursing journal

---

Your dissertation or final assignment is complete: what next?

If you, like the characters in this book, have now completed your evidence-based practice healthcare dissertation/final project or evidence-informed decision-making assignment and you are quite pleased with your grade, what is your next step?

Many nurses believe that writing a paper or article for publication is something that only academics have skills to complete. This is a wrong assumption as there is no mystery attached to writing a paper for publication. It is a skill that anyone with the right amount of determination and application can acquire. All nurses whose work brings them into contact with patients in clinical practice

This chapter is based on an earlier chapter by John Fowler and Colin Rees.

How to Write Your Nursing Dissertation, Second Edition.
Edited by Alan Glasper and Diane Carpenter.
© 2021 John Wiley & Sons Ltd. Published 2021 by John Wiley & Sons Ltd.
Companion website: www.wiley.com/go/glasper/nursingdissertation2e

can be helped to write a paper for a nursing journal. In particular, it is the reflective experiences of nurses working in practice environments that often reveal deficits which may help other nurses to deliver better care or avoid unnecessary mistakes. Additionally, such papers can function as a dissemination platform for sharing ideas. However, it is important for authors to follow a systematic approach to writing a scholarly journal paper as this helps provide a structure that contains key messages and ideas for potential readers. This also applies to the submission of a conference paper or poster.

However, after completing your final work you have three options.

1. Do nothing: enjoy the well-earned rest. Put your work on the bookshelf and let the dust begin to gather!
2. You can try to adapt your work for publication in a suitable journal. This is quite achievable, although it is not as easy as it might initially appear. You will probably need the equivalent of at least a week's work to convert it into an article that might be suitable for publication. It is important not to simply submit your whole dissertation or assignment in full as journal editors will simply reject it.
3. You can submit an abstract of your work, or an aspect of it, for consideration at a suitable conference. This is also quite achievable. It will take approximately one day's work to complete the abstract and, if accepted for presentation at the conference, about another three day's work to prepare the conference presentation paper with its accompanying PowerPoint presentation or poster.

The first option is very tempting, particularly after working hard for a number of years on your degree/foundation degree. However, we would encourage you to consider either or both of options 2 and 3. The very nature of a degree/foundation degree is the recognition that you have moved beyond being a student. You now have something to share; something to teach others in your discipline. By virtue of finishing your degree/foundation degree you have demonstrated not only commitment to your subject but also that you can manage time and complete work to a deadline. Importantly, many students and trainee nursing associates complete their degrees whilst at the same time working clinically and maintaining family commitments. So why stop just because your degree is finished?

Motivation

So what is the first and most important step in getting your work ready for a conference presentation or publication in a journal? It is not the quality of the critical analysis or the general quality of the writing within your dissertation/final assignment. Neither is it the grade you received from the university.

Whilst these are important factors in academic writing and are relevant in published work and conference presentations, they are not the most important factor in moving your work on from completion to potential conference presentation or publication. The most important factor in getting your work more widely recognised is your drive or motivation to take it forward. If you do not really want to get your work more widely acknowledged, then the first knock-back will stop you and your work will remain on the bookcase gathering dust.

So what motivates and drives people to publish their work or present it at a conference, to put in that additional effort?

For some of you it may be part of your role. If you fail to achieve a certain number of publications or conference publications, then your job is in jeopardy. As you can imagine, this is a strong motivator. It is one for example that drives most research nurse academics in university departments. University departments are rated on the quality and quantity of research conferences and publications and this rating attracts considerable funding, hence the drive.

For others, the motivation for taking your work forward is that you want your CV to reflect this level of work and achievement. If you intend applying for more senior roles, such as a clinical nurse specialist, a nurse consultant or a university lecturer, you will be at an advantage if you have conference presentations and publications on your CV. If we were interviewing anyone who had completed a dissertation-based degree or final assignment, we would almost certainly be asking what they subsequently did with their work and the candidate who answers positively is at a great advantage.

Another factor that may motivate you is a simple ambition to present at a national conference or publish in a professional journal, maybe for your family or, often, just to prove to yourself that you can do it. It's a great feeling to see your name on a conference programme or in a journal article.

Some of you who work in specialist areas will have an aspect of practice that you have developed as part of your dissertation/final assignment and you wish to share that with others because you feel very strongly about the subject. What better way than at a conference of people all interested in that particular area of practice.

Conference poster or abstract and presentation at a conference

> **Scenario**
>
> Charlotte has been invited to an end-of-course student conference to present the development and results of her audit tool which was part of her final assignment. She is thrilled but somewhat nervous as there will be 100 people in the audience!

Writing a conference abstract

This is the first and most important step in presenting your work at a conference. There are many nursing conferences each year covering all varieties of clinical specialties. Whatever your subject, you can be sure there is a conference that would welcome a well-constructed abstract regarding your potential paper. This section considers the following aspects of writing a conference abstract:

- choosing the right conference;
- local, national or international conference;
- presenting all or some of your work;
- following the conference committee's abstract guidelines and general structure of the abstract;
- formulating the title and creating interest;
- submission procedure.

Choosing the right conference

A large number of nursing and healthcare conferences are held each year, covering a wide variety of subject themes: clinical specialty, education, research, reflective practice, and an array of alternative aspects of healthcare. Some conferences are very local, organised by a hospital Trust and targeting the local population or, as in the case with Charlotte, a student conference organised by her university nursing studies department. Others are nationally focused and others are international. So which one is right for you? Unlike potential publications to a journal, with conference abstracts you can submit the same or a very similar abstract to different conferences. However, this is not to be recommended. It is far better to research the various conferences, assess them according to various criteria and then make a focused abstract application. So what sort of criteria should you be exploring when considering which conference to submit your abstract to? Consider the following.

1. What date is the conference? Would you be free to attend the conference? This sounds obvious and very 'non-academic' but it is always the first thing to consider. The conference advert for abstracts usually comes out about 10 months prior to the actual conference, but even with that notice you may have something more important in your diary. So make sure you are free to attend the conference and then pencil that date in your diary.
2. Is the conference call for papers asking for subjects that relate to your final work topic? If not, could some aspect of your work be adapted to one of the themes of the conference.
3. Is your evidence-based practice healthcare dissertation/final project or evidence-informed decision-making assignment at the right sort of level

for that particular conference? If you have undertaken a relatively small study in one ward using six interviews, then it is unlikely that the International Conference on Advanced Nursing Research would consider your work. Choose a conference that appears to want your style and level of dissertation. If you are unsure then discuss it with a more experienced colleague who may have been to similar conferences.

4. Where is the conference and would you be able to get funding to attend. You are more likely to get support and funding to attend a conference that is being held 30 miles away, is for one day only and costs £50 to attend rather than for an international conference on the other side of the world, lasting four days and costing over £1000. Most conferences will expect presenters to pay the conference fee and cover their own travelling and accommodation costs.

Local, national or international conference

As you can see from the above, the implications of applying to present at an international conference are significant in terms of cost and travel. If you have undertaken a funded research project, then the cost of results dissemination in terms of conference presentations may have been incorporated into the costing of the research. Other people search the various adverts that appear in the nursing and healthcare journals that offer support for international travel. Occasionally, your local Trust or employer will have special trust funds that have been set aside from legacies to support such travel. It is certainly worth exploring the various options for funding.

Presenting all or some of your dissertation or final project/assignment

Such student work, but especially dissertations, normally has sections on underpinning literature, methodology, sampling technique, data analysis, findings, conclusions and implications for practice. Final projects or assignments may contain plans for or design of an audit. A conference presentation or a poster presentation does not need to cover all of these. Indeed it would be very difficult to do justice to all these in the standard 10 or 20 minute slot that most conferences allocate to such verbal presentations. However, your abstract should give a brief overview of these aspects and then identify the particular focus of your presentation. If you have a lot of data that can be analysed from different perspectives, then you may choose to focus on one particular area for a specific conference, for example age, gender, ethnicity, grade of staff, hospital versus community, and so on.

Following abstract guidelines

Each conference will publish guidelines regarding the structure, content and submission details for the conference abstract. It is very important that you follow the specific guidelines exactly. They generally give you a word limit of approximately 500 words and ask for details which require you to do the following.

1. Identify where your presentation fits into the structure and sub-themes of the conference as presented in their guidelines.
2. Present the theoretical and clinical background which gives context to your work.
3. Identify the methodology or the style of your study, for example 'a survey of 300 staff nurses from one Trust using purposive sampling to represent all wards'.
4. Identify the way in which the data were or are to be analysed.
5. What are the objectives of the study?
6. What if any are the interim findings?
7. Then return to the bigger picture as to how your findings might inform the theoretical and clinical areas identified in the first section.

Formulating the title and creating interest

Conference abstracts, by their very nature, often appear factual but dull. The abstract that you submit, if accepted, will be the one that appears in the conference programme and the one that the conference delegates will use to make their choice of which presentations to attend. This needs to be borne in mind when writing your initial abstract. You have a very limited number of words, so use them to achieve two main objectives: firstly, to convey the quality of the presentation and, secondly, to instill a little intrigue in the reader's mind. You can use the title quite effectively to do this. Review the following examples for ideas.

- Stress levels of clinical nurses: burn out or fade out!
- Nursing leadership: are we herding sheep?
- Advanced nursing skills: the developing role of the Nursing Associate.

Notice how you can use the title to convey precise meaning and also present it in a way that makes people want to read the abstract and the subsequently attend the presentation.

Submission procedure

The submission of your conference abstract is usually electronic. The guidelines are very helpful but must be followed exactly, particularly adhering to the submission dates. Normally you receive an automated response saying your abstract has been received.

Members of the organising committee will review all the abstracts submitted. Normally, each abstract is given to two members of the committee who both make an independent assessment of its potential to be included in the conference. They will use some or all of the following criteria.

- Does the abstract conform to the published guidelines for the conference?
- Is it written and presented at a level consistent with the conference standing and reputation?
- Does the information appear valid and reliable?
- Does the abstract offer a new perspective on an established theory or practice?
- Does the abstract present new knowledge?
- Have there been a number of other similar abstracts covering the same topic?

Scenario

After Sam completed his master's dissertation he submitted an abstract for a local conference and eight weeks later received confirmation of its acceptance. He was both pleased and at the same time anxious as he now had to write his presentation.

Chapter 21

Writing your conference presentation

Congratulations! Your conference abstract has been accepted; now you must write your conference presentation. The good news is that you normally have about four or five months between being notified that your abstract has been accepted and having to actually prepare your presentation. There are two ways that people prepare their presentations.

1. Some people write out verbatim exactly what it is they want to say. They time it to see how long it is going to take during many practice sessions and adjust content accordingly. They produce several pages of notes, often with accompanying PowerPoint images. The presentation has them reading word for word their prepared 'lecture'. The advantage of this is that they cover exactly what they intend to cover; if they are nervous they just have to read their notes and there is no risk of them 'drying up'. The disadvantage of this, as we all know, is that this sort of presentation, even by the most learned people, is quite boring for the listener, so-called 'death by PowerPoint'. The most interesting presentations use very simple slides, and there are some basic rules for using PowerPoint slides: firstly 'keep it simple' and secondly 'avoid putting too much text on one slide'.

2. A second option is to prepare a number of trigger points; these can be PowerPoint slides or any other form of 'prop' and then talk through each of the trigger points without using notes. Some people use photographs or diagrams to give them an aide memoire of what they want to say. To do this successfully you need to know your subject well and be confident enough to know you will not collapse into a nervous and shaking wreck in front of the audience. The other disadvantage of this style is that it is difficult to keep to time, but the advantage is that your presentation is usually far more interesting, conveying not only information but passion and interest as well.

Pick the option that will work for you. If it helps, rather than seeing them as two distinct options, view them as a continuum and construct your presentation somewhere in the middle. Whatever style you choose, make sure you prepare thoroughly.

Preparing a poster presentation

Poster presentations are designed to allow presenters to summarise their work concisely and attractively in order to help publicise it and generate discussion. Such posters may be configured as a mixture of text, tables, graphs and pictures or photographs. Poster sizes vary but the commonest, and that which is used for student presentations, is one which fits onto a standard flip chart easel (65 cm by 95 cm). Conference committees will look for posters of good quality not simply drawn on a thin sheet of flipchart paper. Most universities will have a print centre where posters can be professionally finished at low cost. In 2020, the average cost of a laminated poster was £23.

In practice, many posters are dull and unengaging with text which is too small, confusing layouts and inappropriate colour schemes. Most universities have webpages offering advice on how to prepare a poster or PowerPoint presentation.

Posters are widely used across nursing and other healthcare conferences and feature as part of their programme. At such a conference, the presenter will normally be stood by their poster during the allocated poster presentation periods. This allows the presenter to interact with the other participants and share their work with them. Such academic posters aim to summarise

Chapter 21

Scenario

Alisha is delighted that she has been invited to give a poster presentation at the end of the Nursing Associate course graduation ceremony which aims to highlight the academic achievements of the trainees. Her personal tutor has told Alisha that she can cite this presentation on her CV.

student work concisely and attractively in order to help publicise it and generate discussion.

Writing a paper for publication

> **Scenario**
>
> Sue and Sam have decided that they want to try to publish aspects of their dissertations in a nursing journal. They are tempted to just send off their entire dissertations to the journal that they subscribe to, but is this the best way forward?

The need to plan

Healthcare professionals, particularly clinically based nurses, tend to be very action orientated people; they see something that needs doing and they get on and do it. These are admirable qualities but ones that need just a little holding back if you are to achieve successful publication of your evidence-based practice healthcare dissertation/final project or evidence-informed decision-making assignment. It is not just a matter of sending off your entire work to a journal because this will almost certainly result in a rejection letter. Think of it like planning a patient's care: a little time spent assessing needs and planning the way forward will produce better-quality and more efficient practice and patient care. It is the same with a paper for publication.

Firstly, you need to spend some time assessing the various journals and deciding which one is suitable for your work. Then you need to find, read and implement the authors' guidelines; this will help you produce a better-quality article in a more efficient way. It will produce an article which is much more likely to be accepted for publication than if you had just jumped in and started writing without doing that preparation. The first thing to do is to make yourself familiar with a few copies of the journals that are relevant to your dissertation. Just flick through a few different journals and you will note the general style and variations in what they publish. Each journal is different.

Reviewing the guidelines: what will they tell you?

- *General advice.* This includes the type of article that the journal publishes and the particular readership it targets. It will give you advice about headings, use of boxes, the referencing technique required and general layout of the article. Have a look at the *British Journal of Nursing*'s 'Guidance for Authors'; these are particularly useful and can be found at https://www.magonlinelibrary.com/page/authors/guidance.

- *Article structure.* This includes the word length, the type of headings required, the style of language and the identification of key words. These vary considerably with different journals.
- *Specialist journal advice.* Journals which target a particular topic will often have quite specific advice. For example, the *Journal of Clinical Nursing* has a large section on ethical guidelines (https://onlinelibrary.wiley.com/page/journal/13652702/homepage/forauthors.html).
- *Different types of papers.* Some journals are very specific regarding how particular papers are presented. The *Journal of Advanced Nursing*, for example, has different guidelines on eleven types of papers it publishes including 'systematic reviews', clinical trials, concept analysis and discussion papers (http://www.journalofadvancednursing.com/default.asp?file=authorinfo).

Do not let this important planning stage of writing dampen your enthusiasm for publication. A little time spent choosing the appropriate journal and following their advice is time well spent. As a general rule the journal that you find most useful and interesting to read is the journal you should aim to publish your first article in.

Creating interest

Your dissertations and final projects/assignments have been written according to certain university standards and criteria. Your academic supervisor will have read and marked your work because that is their job, not necessarily because they found it intrinsically interesting. You now need to convert your work into something other people will want to read. Think about your own reading habits. Which articles have you looked at in a journal recently and which of those articles, if any, did you go on to actually read? Your responses to these questions will differ to those of your colleagues but underpinning all the responses will be 'those that appeared interesting to me'. Consider what drew you to look at certain articles? It may be some or all of the following.

- The title: is the title intriguing? Is the topic one in which I am professionally or clinically interested? Is this a subject that is currently in the news? Does the title suggest that I will be able to understand the content of the full article? If not I will probably ignore it.
- The presentation: is the article one big block of writing? Or is it broken up with headings, boxes, diagrams and possibly pictures?
- What do the headings say? Do they provoke interest?

Whether you do this consciously or not, you will be making similar judgements about each of the articles you look at and you will carry out that evaluation in about ten seconds. If during this initial scan something rings positive, then you will stop scanning and pay more attention. You will begin to selectively read bits of the article. It is unlikely that at this stage you will start at the first sentence and read every single sentence in order until you reach the end. For some it goes something like this.

Start with the subtitle: the phrase that follows the main title and which gives you a bit more information about the article.

An examination of the paper abstract: the collection of sentences right at the beginning that is meant to sum up the article, usually about 250 words. But many readers skip reading the abstract if the first sentence does not capture them.

At this stage many readers will look in more detail at the boxes and pictures and scan the sections again to see if there is a particular part of the article that appeals more to them than others. Many nurses always read those short patient case studies that are often presented in boxes.

If at this stage a reader is convinced that this article has something more for them, they will read the conclusion and will look at who has written it and make judgements as to what perspective they are coming from.

Finally and perhaps only rarely will a reader return to the beginning and read the article through from beginning to end!

Now put yourself in the position of an author – it's the same, but in reverse. Firstly, you want to capture the reader's attention, then you want them to start scanning the article and, finally, you want to draw them into the main body of what you are saying. One way of doing this once you have written your article is to put it to one side for a few days and then look at it again, but this time from a reader's perspective; if it does not look interesting, then refine it.

Targeting the right journal

In contemporary healthcare there is now a range of electronic web-based new journals – some good, some ugly, and some very bad with a specific intention of charging you a lot of money for publication. There are an enormous number of journals out there to which you could potentially submit an article. How do you choose which one? Custom and general standards dictate that you do not submit your article to more than one journal at a time, so which one do you adapt your work for? As the time between submission of an article and the editors' response as to rejection or acceptance is on average 8–12 weeks, you cannot afford to keep submitting your work to random journals in the hope that one of them will eventually accept it. In the same way that there are the five 'right' ways to give medication to patients, there are the four 'right' ways to get your evidence-based practice healthcare dissertation/final project or evidence-informed decision-making assignment published in the right journal.

- Right content: is the subject matter appropriate for the journal?
- Right level: what level have you written your work at? Can you adapt it to the journal level?
- Right time: a topical subject is more likely to get accepted than one they have just run a series on.
- Right style: you need to adapt your writing style to that of the journal.

As a general rule, nursing and healthcare-related journals target one of the following areas.

- A variety of clinical issues for all types of nurses, for example *British Journal of Nursing*.
- A specialist medical focus, for example *Comprehensive Child and Adolescent Nursing* (an international nursing journal).
- A professional organisation's journal covering clinical, research and management, reaching the majority of its profession, for example *British Journal of Occupational Therapy*.
- An educational focus, for example *Nurse Education Today*.
- A management focus, for example *Journal of Health Care Management*.
- Weekly topical news and generic issues, for example *Nursing Times* or *Nursing Standard*.

Secondly, journals can be categorised according to their 'research impact' factor. This is the importance that university research funding bodies associate with publications in certain journals. Thus, the *Journal of Advanced Nursing* is recognised as having a higher research impact factor than the *Nursing Times* or the *British Journal of Nursing*.

Finally, journals can be viewed as to their 'readership impact', that is the number of nurses who actually read that journal. So, an article in *Nursing Times* or *British Journal of Nursing* will be read by a far greater audience of clinically based nurses than an article in one of the high-impact research journals.

Thus you are left with choices of where the article from your evidence-based practice healthcare dissertation/final project or evidence-informed decision-making assignment best fits in terms of the specialty of its subject matter, its level of originality and research base as appropriate, who you want to read it and, finally, why you want it published. You may end up writing two articles from your evidence-based practice healthcare dissertation/final project or evidence-informed decision-making assignment for two different journals, one detailing the research base of your work and the second the more general application of your subject to the working staff nurse/nursing associate. If you are still unsure regarding which journal is appropriate for your work, then view the author guidelines for the potential journals and make sure you read some of the article published in these journals so that you are aware of the style and standard required.

One of the main skills of writing for a professional publication is to be organised: assess what, why and how you are going to write, and then submit it to the appropriate journal. As a note of caution, beware of online publications that charge you to publish your work. They may offer easy publication but the financial cost to you is often hidden in the small print.

Adapting an evidence-based practice healthcare dissertation/ final project or evidence-informed decision-making assignment for publication

If Sue and Sam, or you, simply submit your complete evidence-based practice healthcare dissertation/final project or evidence-informed decision-making assignment or even a quickly edited version of it to a journal, then you will almost certainly receive a rejection letter. To understand this you need to think about the difference between an evidence-based practice healthcare dissertation/final project or evidence-informed decision-making assignment and an article in a journal.

What are the characteristics of work written for a university course?
The purpose of an evidence-based practice healthcare dissertation/final project or evidence-informed decision-making assignment is for the student to provide evidence that they demonstrate a degree of understanding of a specific subject. Such work will normally be grounded in the established literature. The student will be expected to show an understanding, discussion and critical analysis of this literature. Usually about 25% of an evidence-based practice healthcare dissertation/final project or evidence-informed decision-making assignment will be reviewing the published literature related to the topic.

What are the characteristics of an article written for professional publication?
- Most articles are between 2000 and 4000 words in length.
- The purpose of an article is to communicate new ideas to someone who may or may not be interested in reading what you have to say.
- It is well presented and paragraphs are usually quite short.
- Headings are used to guide the reader into the subject.
- Approximately 10% of the article will be used to introduce the subject to the non-specialist reader.

Chapter 21

- Approximately 20% of the article will reference the work to the underpinning literature.
- Approximately 70% of the article will be presenting new information or discussion and application of established knowledge.
- An article should be both informative and interesting to read.

The literature review
One of the big differences between writing an evidence-based practice healthcare dissertation/final project or evidence-informed decision-making assignment and converting it for publication is how you use the literature. The percentage of the written work given over to a literature review may be similar, around 20%, but in your article this translates to about 400 words. It is there to show the reader where this article 'fits' in terms of the established body of knowledge on the subject rather than demonstrate the breadth, debate and depth of analysis normally associated with a dissertation. In your article the literature review will normally be short, concise yet thorough. In an international journal it should reflect the international as well as the national literature. It should reflect a historical perspective and then locate the current thinking.

The body of the article
Having established the theoretical underpinning of your work, you then need to identify the body of your article. This should be introduced in a short, concise yet informative way that creates interest in the reader's mind. They should be left knowing the exact details of what you are writing about. Use numbers and precise language; for example, 'a change of practice on a 10 bedded unit after three weeks of planning' or 'the development of a multidisciplinary care pathway for approximately 2000 patients a year with XYZ condition covering both community and hospital treatment'.

Having introduced the main theme of the article, you then need to say what it is that you have done, or discus a different perspective on something that has already been written about. A good article will also have two or three sub-themes that weave through the body of your article. For example, if you were writing about the development of a care plan, you may include as sub-themes some of the following: finance, ethics, change management, infection control, patient satisfaction, and so on. Having two or three sub-themes to your article will help give it structure, depth, continuity and application. These can be drawn together in your conclusion, giving it structure, focus and challenge.

The conclusion and way forward
How does the body of your article relate to the underpinning literature? What themes have emerged and been developed? How does this impact on

Chapter 21

practice? What are the challenges in taking this work forward? What are your views?

You can begin to see how an article differs from that of your evidence-based practice healthcare dissertation/final project or evidence-informed decision-making assignment; whilst they both have a foundation of evidence as their base, their structure and presentation differ.

This chapter has been specifically designed to help people like you write scholarly articles for publication in healthcare science journals. A comprehensive model based on 11 steps and detailing the specific architecture expected for a journal is suggested for the writing of a range of papers (see Chapter 23). This is commensurate with the recognised style of a number of academic journals. A published paper describing this model in depth can be found on the student resource website.

What will you do with your evidence-based practice healthcare dissertation/final project or evidence-informed decision-making assignment?

At the beginning of this chapter we presented you with three choices for you and your dissertation: put it on the shelf and let it and possibly you gather dust; or look for a conference presentation/poster presentation within it; or adapt it or part of it for publication. Over the years we have worked with many nurses and allied healthcare staff, helping them to publish an idea or a topic from their dissertation. None of those people have found it easy, and none of those people have been given time off to write that article. The reason those people have succeeded is not because they are cleverer than others, or that their work was at distinction level, it was because they were determined and hard working. Publication is about focus, effort and hard work. That is why a CV that includes conference/poster presentations and publications as well as your clinical experience and expertise is so important when it comes to senior roles and your promotion – it demonstrates not only knowledge but application, commitment and hard work. Do not let the dust settle on your scholarly achievement!

For further resources for this chapter visit the companion website at
🖳 **www.wiley.com/go/glasper/nursingdissertation2e** where you
will find the published paper on how to write a paper for publication and a
PowerPoint presentation on writing for publication

Chapter 22 Reflecting on your evidence-based practice healthcare dissertation/final project or evidence-informed decision-making assignment journey

Justine Barksby
De Montfort University, Leicester, UK

Scenario

Alisha, Charlotte, Sue and Sam are all required to complete their evidence-based practice healthcare dissertation/final project or evidence-informed decision-making assignment with a reflective section. How they do this will vary based on the nature of their individual projects.

Reflection

Reflection has become a tool utilised extensively in healthcare in recent years, particularly in healthcare education. The benefits of reflection are so widely recognised it is now a requirement for nurses as part of their revalidation with the Nursing and Midwifery Council (2019), with nurses requiring five written reflective accounts and a reflective discussion. These benefits primarily focus on learning from an experience. Ingram and Murdoch (2019) define reflection as the process of making better sense of an event, enabling improvements in the future.

Reflection in nursing enables understanding of 'self' in the context and application of theory to practice. Such reflection is a good way to explore your *individual* and *unique* experiences of writing an evidence-based prac-

This chapter is based on an earlier chapter by Wendy Wigley.

How to Write Your Nursing Dissertation, Second Edition.
Edited by Alan Glasper and Diane Carpenter.
© 2021 John Wiley & Sons Ltd. Published 2021 by John Wiley & Sons Ltd.
Companion website: www.wiley.com/go/glasper/nursingdissertation2e

tice healthcare dissertation/final project or evidence-informed decision-making assignment because reflection is a method by which we can make sense of a situation or experience – good or bad – and begin to understand how we have learned because of (or in spite of) the situation or experience. Reflection should be a purposeful activity which allows us to engage, learn and develop in order to change and improve future practice.

Reflection is a process of self-development and experts on the process of reflection often talk about the 'self', 'self as nurse', 'self as student', and so on. Reflection can help us demonstrate what we have learnt about our 'self' during the evidence-based practice healthcare dissertation/final project or evidence-informed decision-making assignment – what were the good points and what went not so well. Reflection is not just about celebrating success (although that can be part of it) nor should it be just about focusing on any negatives, it should include both. In short, a reflection tells the reader your journey. It should not be simply a description however; it needs to have the application of relevant literature. Johns (2003) describes it as 'thinking about thinking'.

The forefather of reflection was John Dewey (1859–1952), a twentieth-century American philosopher and psychologist who was a campaigner for changing the way in which children were taught. Dewey stated:

We do not learn by doing . . . we learn by doing and realising what came of what we did. . .

(Dewey, 1929, cited by Driscoll and Teh, 2001)

As such, Dewey saw education as a process of experience that required the application of thought. Schön (1983) identified that nursing as a profession can potentially involve decision-making activities that could be construed as messy; in other words, nurses often find it hard to explain their actions, what they do and why they do it. He described this as *knowing-in-action*. However, when having to undertake a new or complex task, the practitioner has to think about what they are doing while they are doing it; Schön (1983) described this process as *reflection-in-action*.

Reflection-in-action might be when you explain to a colleague what you are doing while undertaking a task, thereby having to explain and justify actions and decisions made. *Refection-on-action* is a process that happens after the event. Reflection-on-action might involve two people sitting down together and formally recalling an event, or often in the case of an evidence-based practice healthcare dissertation/final project or evidence-informed decision-making assignment it will more likely involve writing your own thoughts on the process of completing it. Refection-on-action is most likely the type you will undertake.

Chapter 22

Frameworks for reflection

Scenario

Alisha and Charlotte are talking about the reflection part of their evidence-based practice healthcare dissertation/final project or evidence-informed decision-making assignment. Alisha says, 'I just don't know how to get started with this section.' Charlotte advises her that a framework will help with this.

Many of us use a framework to help guide us when undertaking reflection. This ensures we think about all relevant points and helps us avoid simply telling a story.

In nursing we are familiar with frameworks to guide our practice; for example, in the nursing process we *assess, plan, implement* and *evaluate* the care we provide to an individual or a group of clients. This framework (Figure 22.1) is often depicted as a cyclical process.

Frameworks are often called models, but basically they are methods which are designed to help us structure our thoughts and actions. We use frameworks in nursing to ensure that the care we give is based on sound clinical judgement. Likewise, when we reflect we are making a judgement of ourselves in relation to an experience, in this case writing your evidence-based practice healthcare dissertation/final project or evidence-informed decision-making assignment.

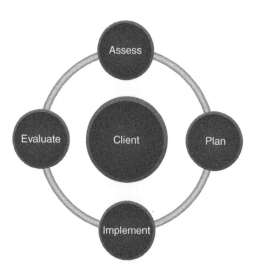

Figure 22.1 The nursing process.

> **Scenario**
>
> Alisha says, 'They sound helpful but how do I choose the right framework or model of reflection?'

There are many models of reflection but no right one; often it is best to choose a model that seems to fit with who you are as a person and how you like to think. The model you choose should make you really think about what you have learnt from writing your evidence-based practice healthcare dissertation/final project or evidence-informed decision-making assignment. Some models are quite simple, others are more complex. The more complex the model, the deeper you can explore your thoughts and, in doing so, the learning you have gained from the experience can also be critical and more analytical.

Gibbs (1988) reflective cycle
One commonly used model is the Gibbs (1988) reflective cycle. This is a six-phase framework (Figure 22.2) that can be used to learn from an experience. The framework's phases each have an underpinning question that you could ask yourself and each of the phases could be used as headings within the final chapter of your evidence-based practice healthcare dissertation/final project or evidence-informed decision-making assignment.

> **Scenario**
>
> Sue and Sam are discussing their reflection sections. Sue looks at the Gibbs cycle and says 'I don't get how it fits with my dissertation'. So Sam draws out the cycle so that it fits the circumstances of Sue's final chapter (Figure 22.3).
>
> Sue notices that Sam has not included 'description' in his drawing. Sam explains that the description element could be the introduction of this chapter, the way in which Sue begins the chapter and explains to her supervisor what this chapter is about.
>
> 'I think I am getting this. . .', says Sue.

Johns (1997) model of structured reflection
Another model of reflection is Johns (1997) as illustrated in Johns (2003) (Figure 22.4). Johns' model integrates Carper's (1978) fundamental ways of knowing to provide guided cues from which reflection can take place and the practitioner can begin to interpret, critically analyse and understand the situation. Carper's (1978) 'Fundamental patterns of knowing in nursing' is based

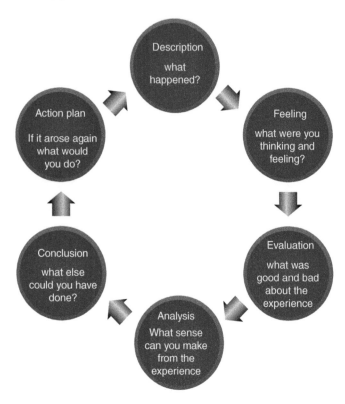

Figure 22.2 The Gibbs reflective cycle. Source: based on Gibbs (1988). © 1988, Oxford University Press.

on how, as nurses, we know what we know about ourselves as practitioners; it is the knowledge that informs what we do in our day-to-day practice.

Aesthetic knowledge is concerned with the 'art' of this situation. Our ability to feel empathy, and in many ways this knowing, is grounded in our subjective reaction to what we see and how we feel about it. So in the case of your evidence-based practice healthcare dissertation/final project or evidence-informed decision-making assignment, this knowing is how you felt about your project.

Scenario

Sam decided to use Johns' model for his reflection. So we know that he was trying to achieve his MSc, but what did he really feel? Apprehensive, out of his depth, confused? Or maybe he felt excited, confident or inspired?

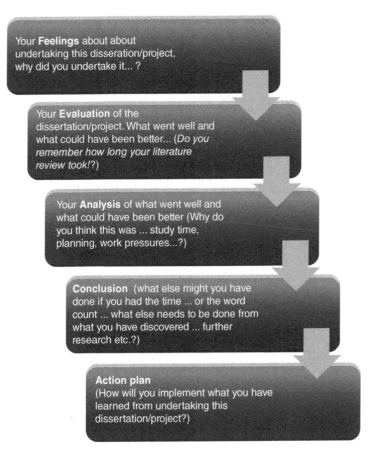

Your **Feelings** about about undertaking this disseration/project, why did you undertake it... ?

Your **Evaluation** of the dissertation/project. What went well and what could have been better... (*Do you remember how long your literature review took!*?)

Your **Analysis** of what went well and what could have been better (Why do you think this was ... study time, planning, work pressures...?)

Conclusion (what else might you have done if you had the time ... or the word count ... what else needs to be done from what you have discovered ... further research etc.?)

Action plan (How will you implement what you have learned from undertaking this dissertation/project?)

Chapter 22

Figure 22.3   Gibbs reflective cycle applied to the final reflective chapter of Sue's dissertation.

Personal knowledge is our attempt to understand ourselves; we need to explore how our cultural and life experiences have shaped us and what judgements we may make about situations or people as a result of these experiences. Personal knowing is about what makes us who we are.

Scenario

For Sam this is what made him decide to undertake this study in the first place. Why did he want to be a nurse with a master's degree and what influenced this decision? What was it about his personal experiences that made him choose to look at the topic he did for his dissertation?

Write a description of the experience
• What are the significant issues I need to pay attention to?

Reflective cues:

Aesthetics
• What was I trying to achieve?
• Why did I repond the way I did?
• What were the consequences of that for: the patient, others myself?
• How was this person feeling?
• How did I know this?

Personal
• How did I feel about the situation?
• What internal factors were influencing me?

Ethics
• How did my actions match my beliefs?
• What factors made me act in incongruent* ways? (* *he means different Sue*)?

Empirics
• What knowledge should have informed me?

Reflexivity
• How does this connect with previous experience?
• What would the consequences be of alternative actions for: the patient, others, myself?
• How do I now *feel* about this experience?
• Can I support myself and others better as a consequence?
• Has this changed my way of knowing?

Figure 22.4 Johns (1997) model of structured reflection. Source: based on Johns (2003).

Ethical knowledge is about our morals and the principles we hold and is linked to personal knowing. Ethics of a situation requires us to explore the extent to which we value and respect individuals or ourselves.

Empirical knowledge relates to evidence, literature and theories that support practice. For Sam this element should be the easiest to describe, as this

Scenario

Sue asks Sam 'Why did you want to look at the topic you chose?' and then a difficult question 'Did you suspect that the care that was being given was not as good as it could be?'

will relate to the evidence he has established and the knowledge he has gained from undertaking his dissertation.

Reflexivity refers to your position in this work, and therefore it is important to acknowledge that the perspective of you, the student, shapes the work.

Scenario

'So', says Sam, 'this is the bit where I summarise all of the above. I'll try not to be too self-conscious but write about . . . me'.

Reflexivity is really the point where Sam can really look at 'Sam the person' and, as Bolton (2005) describes, tell the story of how Sam's dissertation journey has changed his sense of self.

The REFLECT model

Another model available conveniently uses the word 'reflect' as a mnemonic to help us remember each stage. The REFLECT model (Barksby *et al.*, 2015) stands for:

R   RECALL the events

E   EXAMINE our responses

F   Acknowledge FEELINGS

L   LEARN from the experience

E   EXPLORE options

C   CREATE a plan of action

T   Set TIMESCALE

Chapter 22

These can be elaborated as follows.

Stage 1   RECALL the events: a brief overview of the situation on which the person is reflecting. This should consist of the facts, a description of what happened.

Stage 2   EXAMINE our responses: the reflector should discuss their thoughts and their actions at the time of the situation on which they are reflecting.

Stage 3   Acknowledge FEELINGS: the reflector highlights any feelings they experienced at the time of the situation on which they are reflecting.

Stage 4   LEARN from the experience: this stage should highlight what the reflector has learnt from the situation.

Stage 5   EXPLORE options: here the reflector can discuss options for the future if they were to encounter a similar situation or undertake a similar project.

| Stage 6 | CREATE a plan of action: this can be for future theoretical learning or action. |
| Stage 7 | Set TIMESCALES: a time by which the plan outlined in stage 6 will be complete. |

The seven stages ensure that a thorough reflective learning cycle takes place and yet the mnemonic makes it extremely easy to understand and remember.

Borton (1970) model

Borton's model has three stages and although often regarded as a simple model it nonetheless still covers the key areas required for the reflective process. Like REFLECT, it is very easy to remember.

Borton's model consists of the following stages.

- *Stage 1: What?* We are encouraged to discuss what happened (what did you do?).
- *Stage 2: So what?* We are encouraged to explore our thoughts and feelings about the 'what' stage and how we have developed as a result.
- *Stage 3: Now what?* This asks what we may have done differently had we had more time, or know at the beginning what we know now and also what we will do in the future.

Scenario

Alisha decides that as she has less words available to use in her literature review she will use Borton's model so she can write it more succinctly. Charlotte has more words available for this section so is going to choose Gibbs.

Choosing a model

There is no correct model to choose, although your university may advise on a particular one. If your university does not specify which you must use, it is worth looking at a few to see if one appeals to you more than the next.

Some final points on reflection

Reflection is *not*:

- a stick with which to beat yourself or others;
- a descriptive account;
- to be shared if you are uncomfortable/not ready;

- to be shared with those who you do not trust;
- to be criticised.

Instead, reflection should be:

- an opportunity for personal growth and professional development;
- very challenging;
- a compassionate, non-judgemental observation of our own experiences.

Conclusion

There are a plethora of models of reflection (not just the ones included here) and if given a choice it is worth exploring the one that suits you the best. The process of reflection should enable you to analyse and clarify experiences in order to develop and, importantly, should contain a forward-looking stage that helps you improve for the future. Reflection is a useful way to complete a project and a useful skill within nursing.

References

Barksby, J., Butcher, N. and Whysall, A. (2015) A new model of reflection for clinical practice. *Nursing Times*, **111** (34–35), 21–23.

Bolton, G. (2005) *Reflective Practice*, 2nd edn. Sage Publications, London.

Borton, T. (1970) *Reach, Touch, and Teach: Student Concerns and Process*. McGraw-Hill, New York.

Carper, B.A. (1978) Fundamental patterns of knowing in nursing. *Advances in Nursing Science*, **1** (1), 13–23.

Dewey, J. (1929) *Experience and Nature*. Grave Press, New York.

Driscoll, J. and Teh, B. (2001) The potential of reflective practice to develop individual orthopaedic nurse practitioners and their practice. *Journal of Orthopaedic Nursing*, **5**, 95–103.

Gibbs, G. (1988) *Learning by Doing: A Guide to Teaching and Learning Methods*. Further Education Unit, Oxford Polytechnic, Oxford.

Ingram, P. and Murdoch, M. (2019) How to reflect on your practice. Nursing in Practice. https://www.nursinginpractice.com/professional/how-to-reflect-on-your-practice/ (accessed 27 December 2019).

Johns, C. (2003) Opening the doors of perception. In: C. Johns and D. Freshwater (eds) *Transforming Nursing through Reflective Practice*. Blackwell Publishing, Oxford.

Schön, D. (1983) *The Reflective Practitioner: How Professionals Think in Action*. Basic Books, New York.

Chapter 22

For further resources for this chapter visit the companion website at
 www.wiley.com/go/glasper/nursingdissertation2e

Chapter 23 **Building the architecture of your dissertation**

Diane Carpenter[1] and Alan Glasper[2]
[1]*University of Plymouth, UK*
[2]*University of Southampton, UK*

Writing your evidence-based practice healthcare dissertation/final project or evidence-informed decision-making assignment

Stage 1: Decimal notation system

Use the decimal notation system, commonly known as the civil service format, to write each section of your work. You will see that this is the system used for all published healthcare policies. Although not compulsory, many students writing evidence-based practice healthcare dissertations/final projects or evidence-informed decision-making assignments find it easier to use the civil service format for delineating the various subsections of their work. Consequently, in Chapter 1 the main heading of an evidence-based practice (EBP) assignment might be:

1   Writers disease (main heading), followed by

1.1   The incidence of Writers disease (smaller heading), and then possibly followed by

1.1.1   Gender differences in Writers Disease (small heading), and so on.

Still in Chapter 1, the next section might be 1.2 The prevalence of Writers disease, with subsections as above. This might then be followed by 1.3 The management of Writers disease, in turn followed by 1.4 The role of government

This chapter is based on an earlier chapter by Alan Glasper and Colin Rees.

How to Write Your Nursing Dissertation, Second Edition.
Edited by Alan Glasper and Diane Carpenter.
© 2021 John Wiley & Sons Ltd. Published 2021 by John Wiley & Sons Ltd.
Companion website: www.wiley.com/go/glasper/nursingdissertation2e

policy in managing Writers disease, 1.5 The role of evidence-based practice in the management of Writers disease, 1.6 Formulating an EBP question pertinent to Writers disease using the PICO framework. This style of formatting can be used throughout the whole evidence-based practice healthcare dissertation/ final project or evidence-informed decision-making assignment; hence, Chapter 2 would follow similarly with 2.1, 2.1.1, and so on, 2.2, 2.3, and so on.

Scenario

Sue does not really understand the decimal notation format of report writing and her friend Sam gives her a good suggestion. He asks her to examine any government healthcare report. Sue accesses one of the National Service Frameworks and suddenly it becomes clear to her!

Stage 2: Searching the literature and sourcing the evidence

Many students find this the most technically difficult chapter to write. It is a formulaic chapter and must include a number of subsections to demonstrate that the student has not simply sourced the papers randomly from the internet. Perhaps because of this, most searching the literature chapters follow the same format. This normally constitutes Chapter 2 of the evidence-based practice healthcare dissertation/final project or evidence-informed decision-making assignment and should include the following.

- Reference to a literature searching method (e.g. Timmins and McCabe, 2005).
- Discussion of a hierarchy of evidence in healthcare. What is best and why?
- Navigating the scholarly databases in selecting evidence. What are the bibliographic databases and which have been used? Students should consider using a table. (The sample dissertation hosted on the companion website of this book at www.wiley.com/go/glasper/nursingdissertation2e provides an example of the chapter architecture required for this element.)
- Searching the literature by hand. Here the student should discuss how hand searching complemented the search of the bibliographic databases.
- Searching the Cochrane database (http://ukcc.cochrane.org/) and other eminent databases, such as the Centre for Reviews and Dissemination hosted by the University of York (http://www.york.ac.uk/inst/crd/) and the Joanna Briggs Institute for Evidence-Based Nursing (http://www.joannabriggs.edu.au/).
- Using grey literature. It is important to include some reference to the use of grey literature in this element of the dissertation.
- Using expert opinions. Students wishing to gain extra insights into the solving of clinical questions are advised to seek opinions from key informant experts, such as clinical researchers, clinical nurse specialists and consultants. Evidence of correspondence with their key informants can be

Chapter 23

alluded to in the text, with letters and emails being placed in one of the appendices if used.

- Using the internet. It is important to give details of how you have used the internet search engines, such as Google, Google Scholar and so on, but you must also discuss their strengths and limitations.
- Using health services benchmarked practice policy publications, such as government health policies, to source additional evidence is always helpful and a useful inclusion for any evidence-based practice healthcare dissertation/final project or evidence-informed decision-making assignment.
- Give details of your database search strategy with key search terms, Boolean logic, wildcards and truncations (students are recommended to consider using a table).

Scenario

All the students have been getting to grips with searching the literature. One of the lecturers has given them a table of an initial search strategy he used for some work on evaluating clown humour for children in hospital.

Databases searched for the clown humour example

- AMED 1985–2005
  Search terms: (Laughter/or clown$ or "Wit and humor"/) AND (child$ or pediatric or paediatric)
- BNI British Nursing Index 1985–2005
  Search terms: (humour/or clown$ or laughter) AND (child$ or pediatric or paediatric)
- CINAHL 1982–2005
  Search terms: (Hospitals, Pediatric/or Child, Hospitalized/) AND (clown$ or laughter)
- EMBASE 1980 to Week 18 2005
  Search terms: (Pediatric hospital/or Child Hospitalization/) AND (clown$ or laughter)
- HMIC Health Management Information Consortia 1983–2005
  Search terms: (Humour/or clown$ or laughter)
- MEDLINE 1966 to April Week 3 2005
  Search terms: (Laughter therapy/or Laughter/or "Wit and humor"/or clown$) AND (Hospitals, pediatric/or Child hospitalized/)
- PsycInfo 1985 to April Week 4 2005
  Search terms (Humor/or clown$ or laughter) AND (hospitalized patients or pediatrics)
- Web of Science 1981–2005
  Search terms: (laughter or clown$) AND (child$ or pediatric or paediatric)

- ASSIA Applied Social Sciences Index and Abstracts 1987–2005
  Search term: clown$
- Index of Theses (including Irish section)
  Search terms: clowns or laughter
- University library catalogue: clowns
- British Library catalogue: (1) clowns and (therapy or hospital*); (2) laughter and (therapy or hospital*)
- Library of Congress: clowns and (therapy or hospital*)
- Southampton City Library: clowns or laughter
- Articlesfirst Database: ArticleFirst Query: kw: therapy and ti: laughter

- It is important to include a table of the inclusion and exclusion criteria applied.
- Prepare a long shortlist of papers that have been identified. Students should consider putting this in a table format with author, title, journal and year of publication, the database, and a brief outline of the study. The final selection of three to five data-driven papers should be double starred (more for postgraduate and PhD dissertations).
- Accurately list, using the Harvard reference system, your final shortlist selection of papers.
- Use the Savage and Callery grid method to display the primary attributes of your selected papers. (A copy of a Savage and Callery grid is available via the web resource which accompanies this book.)

Stage 3: Critical appraisal

In this section of the evidence-based practice healthcare dissertation/final project or evidence-informed decision-making assignment, which is often Chapter 3, students are advised to include sections pertinent to the following.

- What is critical appraisal?
- Types of critiquing tools.
- Selection of the critiquing tool(s).
- Following each step of the tool to critique the selected papers. It is recommended that students critique the papers collectively and not one by one.
- It is important to stress that all critiquing tools require readers to investigate the results or data analysis section of the papers they are appraising. For most undergraduate work this requires a preliminary understanding and description of the statistics used in the papers. For postgraduate dissertations significantly more detail is required.

Chapter 23

Stage 4: Conclusions and implications

The conclusions and implications of the literature critique are usually formatted as a separate chapter and should include:

- details pertinent to the value of the research findings for the student's particular field of practice;
- a table showing the strengths and limitations of the studies should be included in this section;
- a summary of the evidence from each paper critiqued and an assessment of the value of the evidence.

Stage 5: Implementing evidence in practice

In this section (often the final chapter of your work) students are required to consider how evidence can be introduced into practice. They are asked to write about the barriers or impediments that prevent full implementation of evidence in clinical environments. This includes a number of aspects.

- Managing change in clinical practice: some universities require students to consider change theory.
- The role of leadership in the management of change: students are often required to include the work of the Royal College of Nursing (https://www.rcn.org.uk/professional-development/professional-services/leadership-programmes) and The Kings Fund (https://www.kingsfund.org.uk/consultancy-support/organisational-development), which have been at the forefront of leadership and change within healthcare settings.
- Students must consider the barriers to change and, importantly, include fully referenced detail on how to overcome these barriers.

Stage 6: Reflection

Many universities expect students to use a model of reflection in the final aspect of the evidence-based practice healthcare dissertation/final project or evidence-informed decision-making assignment to describe their academic journey.

Stage 7: Using appendices

Although dissertation markers cannot award marks for appendices, they can judge overall student effort through the quality of appendices. The student can use appendices to ensure that the whole is greater than the sum of the parts. The strict word count applied to any student submission does not apply to appendices and students can use them to place important evidence of their overall effort and furthermore allude to this within the text of individual chapters.

> **Scenario**
>
> The students have been contemplating how they can best optimise the appendices facility afforded within the overall submission.
>
> Sue has decided to append a full copy of the critiquing tool she has used and Alisha is considering appending her correspondence with the range of clinical nurse specialists she has written to during her academic journey.

Stage 8: Using the supervisor/tutor

All students writing an evidence-based practice healthcare dissertation/final project or evidence-informed decision-making assignment are advised to use their supervisor wisely, be cognisant of word limits, be fully aware of how the dissertation should be formatted and, importantly, understand the importance of proofreading their work for 'typos' and spelling/grammatical errors.

Stage 9: References

Students can be penalised up to 10% for reference errors. The crime of reference error is an own goal. Best avoided!

Stage 10: Binding

Some universities still expect a fully bound dissertation, although most will now accept an electronic submission of work. If required to provide a bound copy, allow at least five working days for binding. (Hot tip: bind a photocopy of the dissertation rather than a copy from a printer as the process of printing often distorts the pages.)

Stage 11: Gaining an academic extension

Universities are very sympathetic to students who require an extension period to finish their work. This especially applies to students learning beyond registration where job pressure may negatively impact on best-laid temporal plans. All universities have procedures to consider student appeals for mitigation or course work extension. However, students are advised to ask for this ahead of time and not on the day the dissertation is scheduled to be submitted!

Chapter 23

> **Scenario**
>
> It is summertime and the students have just met in the local pub to celebrate their success in being awarded their degrees at the university conferment of awards ceremony. A great result!

Reference

Timmins, F. and McCabe, C. (2005) How to conduct an effective literature search. *Nursing Standard*, **20** (11), 41–47.

For further resources for this chapter visit the companion website at
        www.wiley.com/go/glasper/nursingdissertation2e

Section 7 **Bonus chapters (website only)**

Don't forget to go to www.wiley.com/go/glasper/nursingdissertation for:

- Additional chapters
- Summaries of each chapter in the book
- A range of tools and frameworks
- Sample documents to assist you writing your dissertations/projects/final assignments
- Useful reference links
- Reference lists for each chapter.

Index